Simplified Cardiac Medications

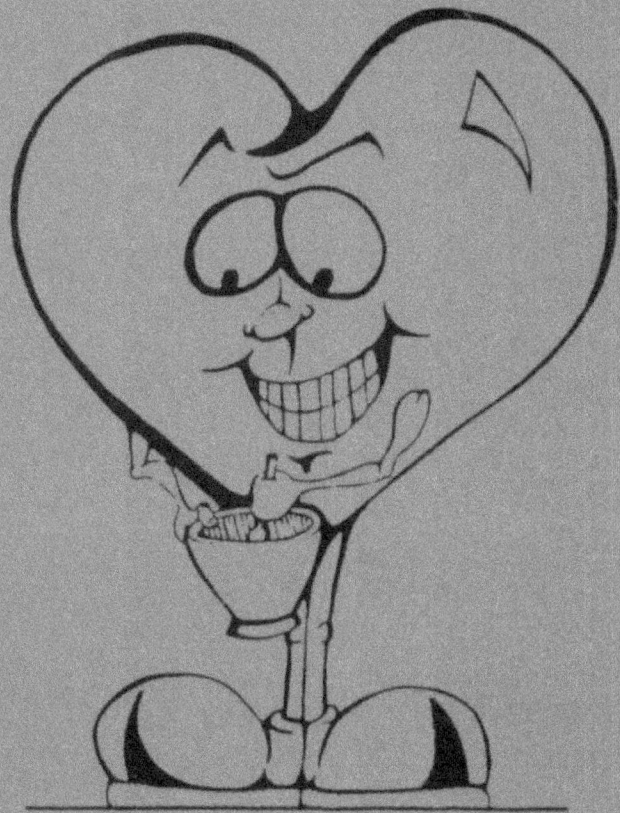

SIMPLIFIED CARDIAC MEDICATIONS

Malcolm Rosenberg, R.N.
Steven Cohn, M.D., F.A.C.C.

To Randie without whose encouragement this would not have been possible. S.C.

To the two new humans in my life since I started on this book, my friend Ian Pearl and my new daughter-in-law Tara & to the new animals in my life, Hydey, Kitty, Bailey, Shadow, Sam and Cali and to Tiny who left my life in that time period. M.R.

Cardiac physiology, pathophysiology and pharmacology are the same material seen from different perspectives. Usually this material is taught in three separate classes, Physiology and pharmacology and the cardio-pulmonary rotation. That is wasting time and losing opportunities to learn. The three subjects should be taught together. That is the whole point of this book.

That is the opportunity of this book and it is the challenge. We do away with the usual linear format of presenting each subject separately. You will see

PHYSIOLOGY PATHOPHYSIOLOGY PHARMACOLOGY,

three traditionally separate threads are interwoven here.

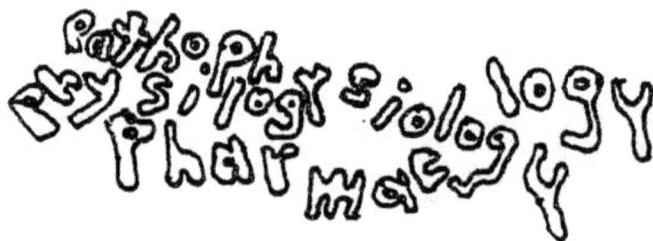

Consequently lot of facts will be repeated and re-repeated. There is no perfect arrangement for a lot of overlapping material.

What this book does not have is things to memorize. There are plenty of other books to look up loading doses and onset, peak and duration. I think that would detract from the reason for this book - to understand how cardiac medications work.

Trust me on this: it won't look like any other text book you've seen.

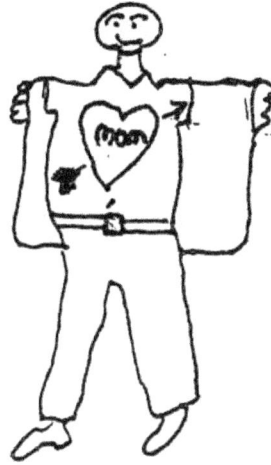

O.K. Let's go.

Adrenaline. What comes to mind when you hear that word? Impending danger. Your heart racing. Your mouth as dry as a bone. That's all correct and much more. That's because adrenaline is a chemical your body produces to give it a huge boost when danger confronts us.

It might surprise you to know that the physiological systems that produce adrenaline comprises most of what this book is about. Just from experiencing a pounding heart rate in stressful situations you can appreciate its strength.

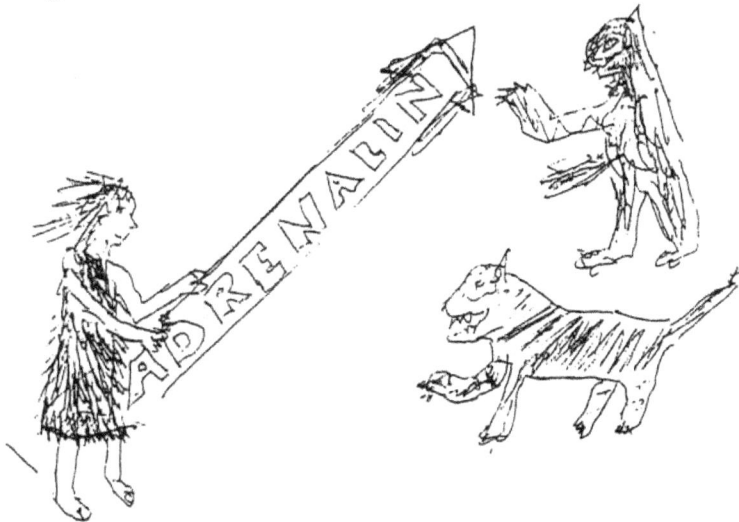

You may have heard it called "fight or flight."
We will be looking at the strength of this system.

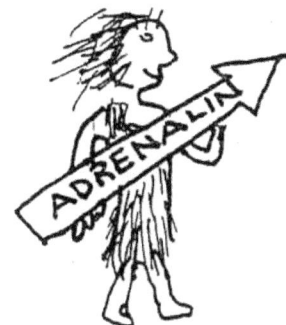

2

We will look at its components.

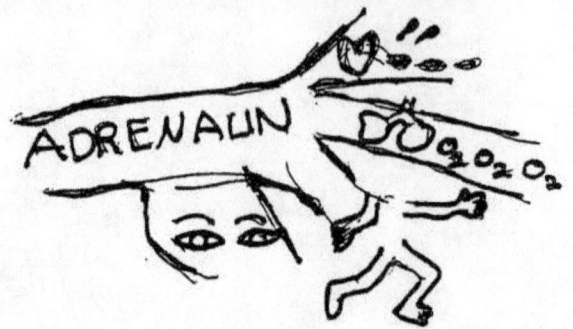

We will look at drugs that stimulate "fight or flight."

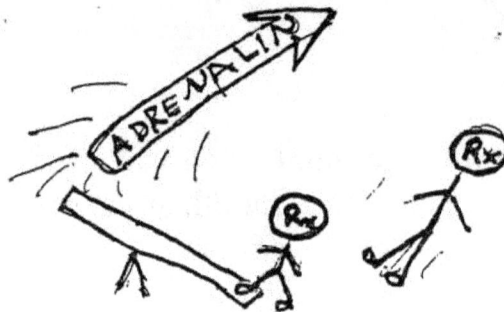

And we will look at drugs that block all or part of it.

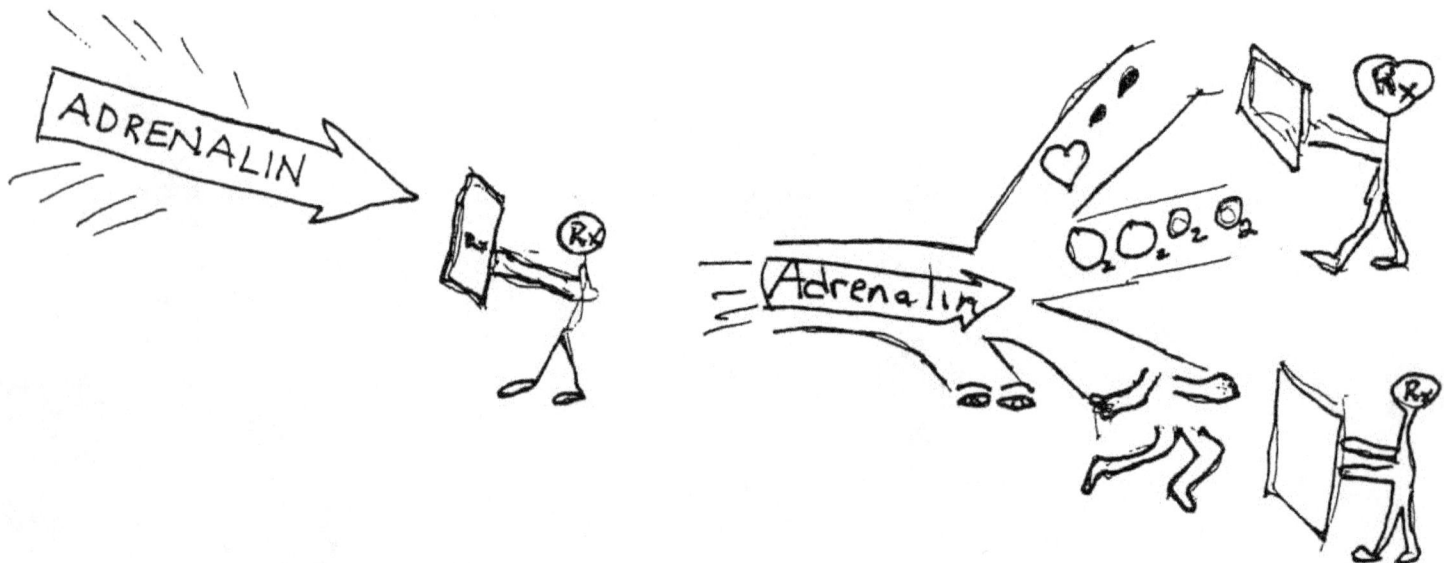

Now to get down to business.

The heart (anatomy) is a muscle that pumps blood (physiology). I will depict the heart by this drawing. There are four chambers, the right atrium, the right ventricle, the left atrium and the left ventricle.

Blood returns to the right atrium from the vena cava. 75% of the blood from both atria drops passively into the ventricles through the tricuspid and mitral valves.

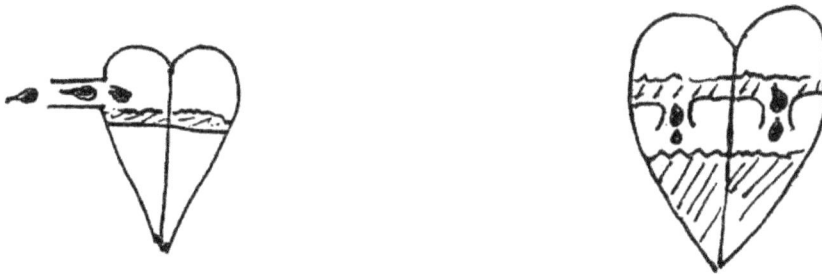

Then the sinus node fires and the electrical charge rushes through the atria and causes them to contract. That contraction squeezes the last 25% of the blood into the ventricles. As the atria contract and mitral and tricuspid valves open further, the ventricles complete their filling

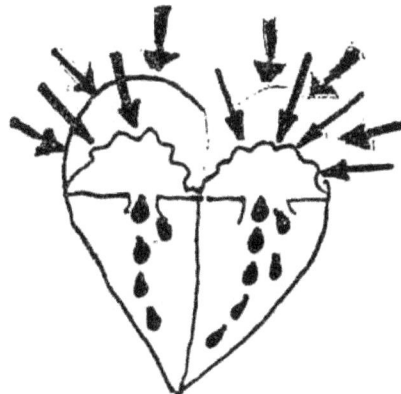

After the atria have both contracted, the charge continues through the AV (atrioventricular) node. It continues along the conduction fibers. In the order of conduction: the bundle of His, the Left and right bundle branches, the Purkinje fibers.

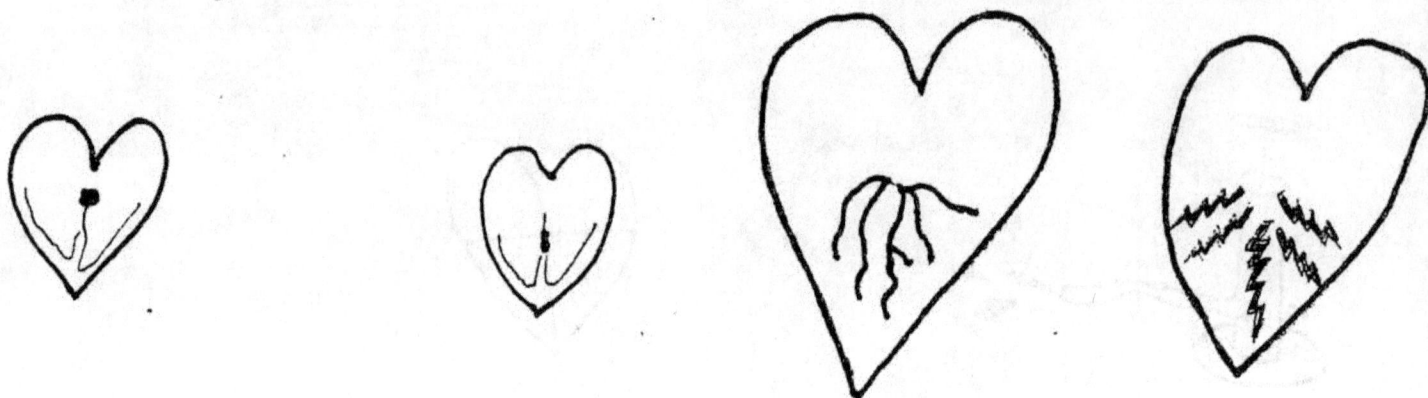

From those numerous fibers the charge spreads through the ventricles causing the ventricular contraction. The ventricular contraction squeezes out most of its blood from the right side into the lungs and from the left into the aorta.

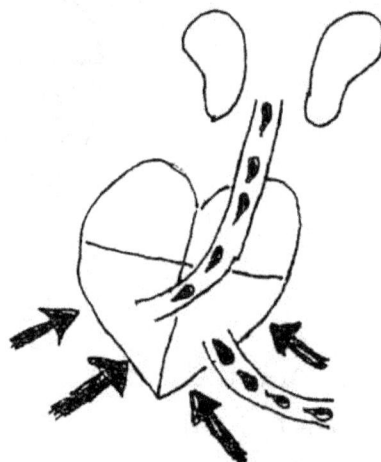

The next 75 pages will explain those last few paragraphs in greater detail. And they will include heart disease and medical response – in other words, cardiac physiology, pathophysiology and pharmacology. It will separate the heart study into three systems: muscular, conduction and circulation.

CARDIAC MUSCLES

You instinctively know that an electrical current causes large muscles to contract. An electrical shock, however small, causes your muscles to uncontrolabley jerk. On the level of an microscopic muscle cell it is the same.

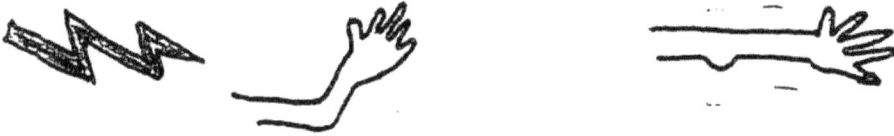

The heart muscle cell contains a certain amount of calcium, sodium and potassium inside the cell (intracellular) and another concentration of calcium, sodium and potassium outside of the cell (extracellular). Muscle contraction requires a sequential series of sodium, potassium and calcium transferred back and forth across the cell membrane. This ionic flow in and out of the cell can be measured electrically. That is known as an EKG.

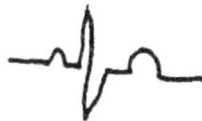

An electrical charge to the muscle cell initiates the contraction. Before the muscle cell is zapped, it is resting and relaxing. The various concentrations of charged ions inside of the cell give it a voltage of –90 millivolts. That is called the resting potential (voltage). When an outside electrical source zaps the cell the voltage goes up. When the voltage inside the cell reaches –70 millivolts things start to happen. –70 millivolts is called the threshold voltage. Threshold means the beginning. When the voltage reaches –70 a cascade of events begins. This cascade is the series of individual changes in each cell that take place when the muscle contracts and then passes it on to the next cell to propagate the contraction.

In the next few paragraphs we will describe this cascade of events. Definitely do not memorize it. In fact you don't even have to understand it unless you are a cardiologist studying for the boards. If you are a cardiologist studying for the boards I would recommend Textbook on Cardiology by Hurst. It is about 2200 pages longer than this and goes into a little more detail. However it does not have the section on medical jokes which this book has.

CARDIAC MUSCLE CONTRACTION

The process of muscle contraction in general and cardiac muscle contraction in particular is a complicated process of myocin and actin fibrils sliding into each other or "interdigitating". Try to use this word frequently when ever you are discussing anything related to the heart.

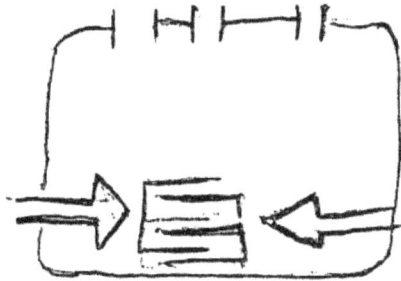

Calcium is an essential ingredient. More calcium generally means stronger and faster contraction. Less calcium generally means slower and weaker contraction.

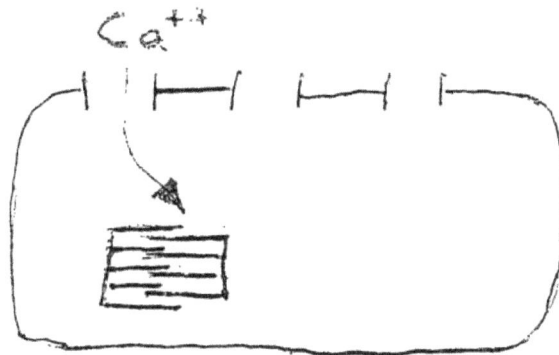

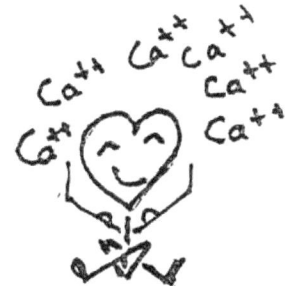

The process is initiated by a very small electrical charge about one tenth of a volt. It is called an "action potential". Try to use that term frequently in any situation.

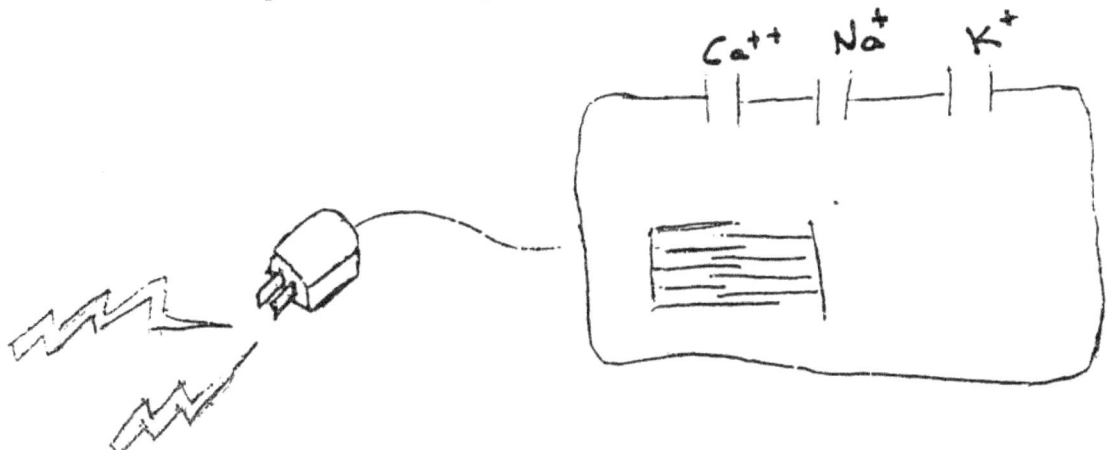

The voltage of a muscle cell at rest is –90 millivolts. When an outside charge increases the voltage to –70 millivolts (remember –70 is more than –90) a series of events is started that cause the muscle cell to contract.

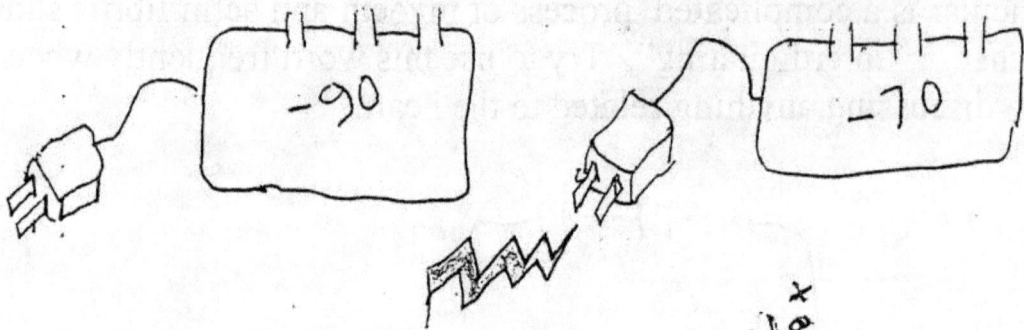

Sodium rushes in through the sodium channels.

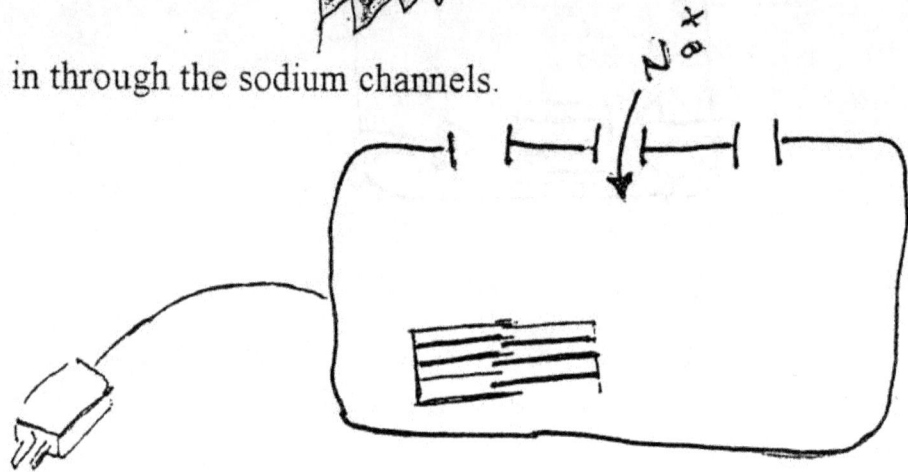

Potassium leaves the cell.

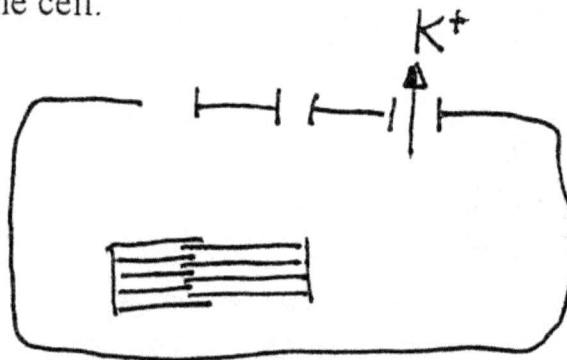

Calcium goes in via the calcium channel.

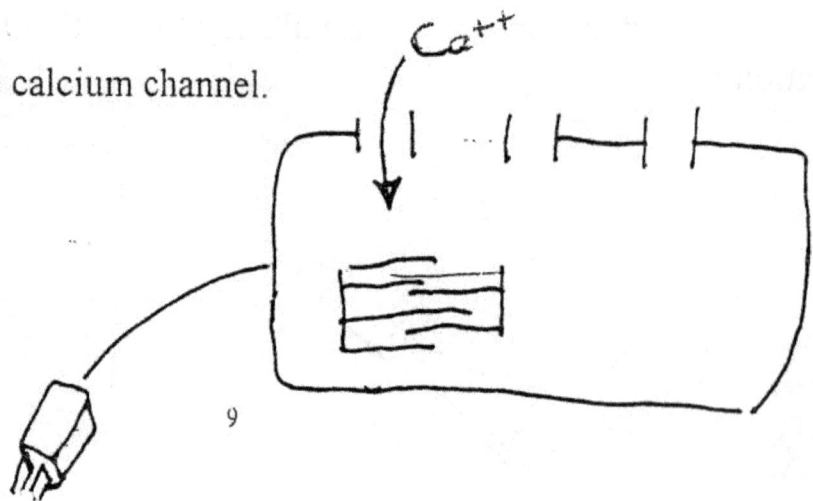

9

It is calcium that facilitates the myocin and actin fibrils to contract (or interdigitate).

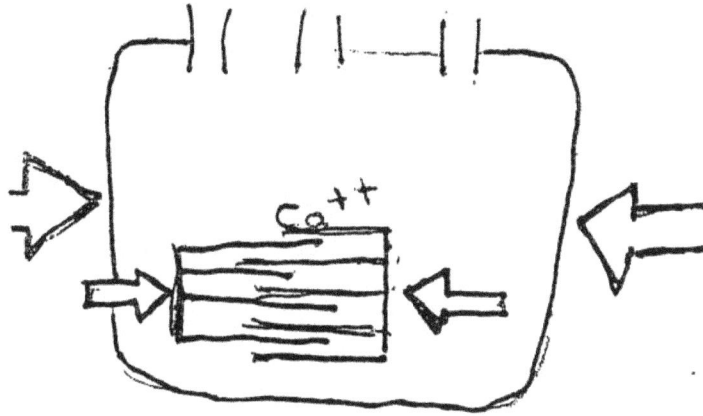

As long as calcium stays on the fibrils the muscle cell remains contracted.

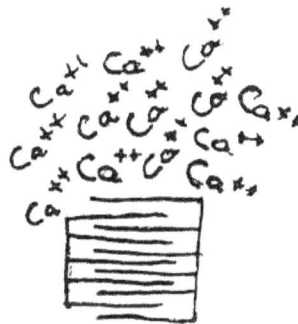

The influx of calcium and sodium ions causes the electric charge (potential) of the cell to reach +10 millivolts (up from −70). +10 volts is enough to start the cycle in an adjacent cell. Remember the calcium and sodium are positive.

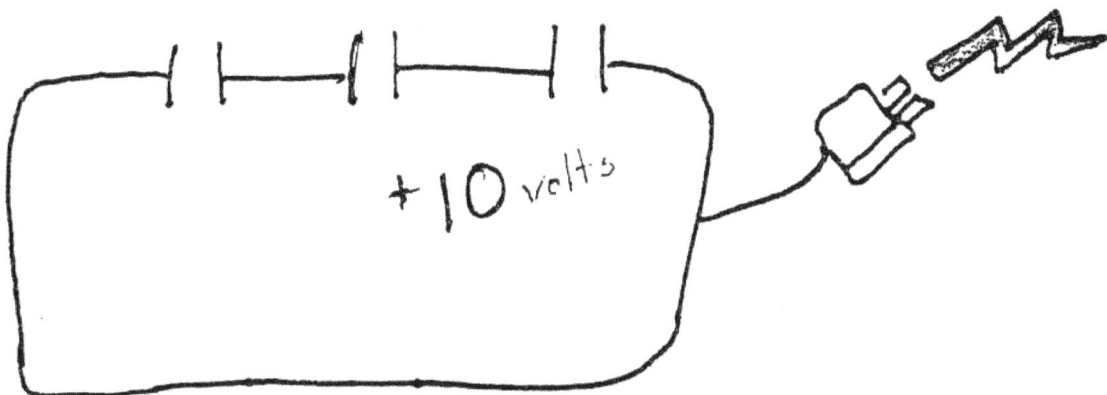

To relax the muscle cell from its contracted state, the calcium must be taken out. The process starts with a pump in each muscle cell called the **"Na+,K+ -ATP"** pump. It pumps the sodium and calcium out and the potassium back in. That restores the muscle cell to its original voltage.

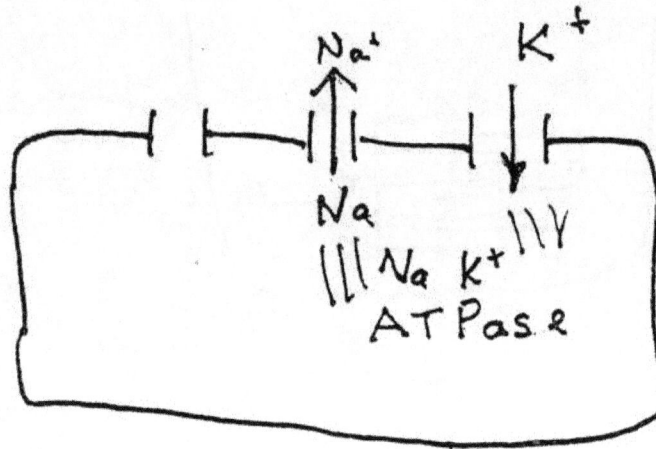

Then the **Na+,K+,-ATPase** pumps in some more sodium to push out the calcium on the myocin and actin fibrils. This causes the "interdigitated" fibrils to come apart or the muscle fibers to relax.

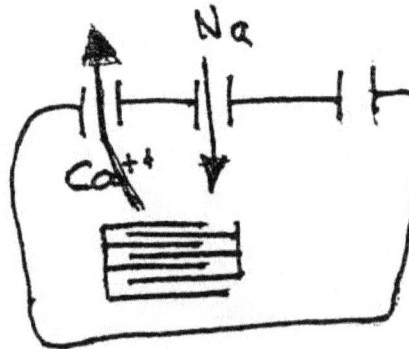

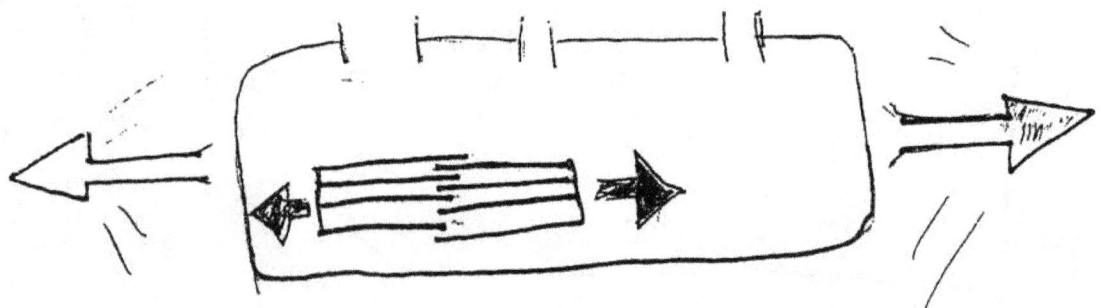

In summary: the SA node (1) starts the sequence of contraction. The cell(2) contracts. After the contraction, it zaps(3) the adjacent cell. Then it returns to its normal configuration(4).

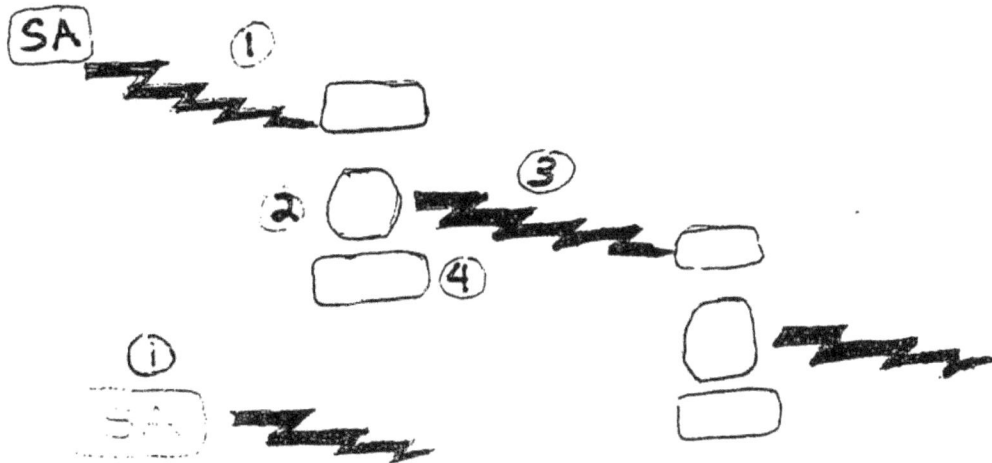

GET READY FOR THE NEXT SECTION – FIGHT OR FLIGHT
(It may appear in the next few pages that we are digressing. No. We are focusing on very powerful drivers on the heart, blood and circulation. They are extremely cogent to the study of cardiac medications. All cardiac medications either enhance or squelch these explosive energy accelerators. So if we can understand the so called fight or flight mechanism, we can understand cardiac medications.

FIGHT OR FLIGHT

The human body has a way of turning on the speed. The **fight or flight** mechanism quickly activate a number of systems that enable the body to fight or fly in stressful situations. When a cave man ran into a saber tooth tiger the cave man had to run away or fight it. The sympathetic nervous system and the adrenergic system do this. It activates target organs to increase their output.

The sympathetic nervous system quickly increases the body's physical output (in a matter of seconds).

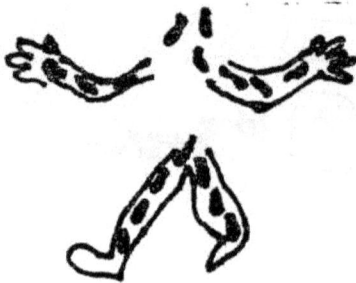

It redirects blood flow to skeletal muscles.

It provides more oxygen. (where target organs are the lungs)

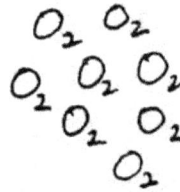

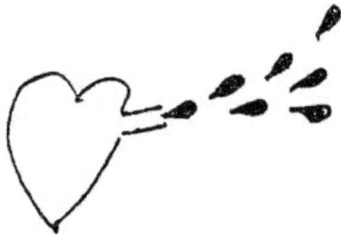

It increases cardiac output. (where The target organ is the heart)

It provides sugar. (where the target organ is the liver)

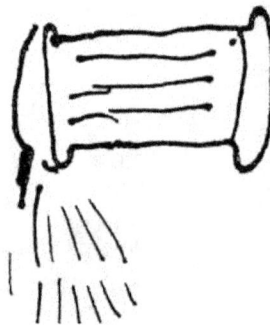

A number of cardiac drugs act on these systems – either inhibiting them or enhancing them. Lets look at how these systems work before we talk about changing them with drugs.

The response to a fight or flight condition begins in the brain – usually a strong emotion like terror triggers the impulse. (1) It travels down the spinal cord along nerve pathways called neurons. (2) The impulse reaches the target organs at a **receptor** site. Here at the end of the neuron is a synapse. The synapse is the connection from the nerve to the target organ. The neurotransmitter (norepinepherine) that will cross over into the target organ is stored in the synapse.(3) the impulse causes one side of the synapse to release the neurotransmitter to the other side on the target organ. The neurotransmitter is norepinepherine which crosses from the neuron side to the target organ side. Norepinepherine is abbreviated "NE." (4)

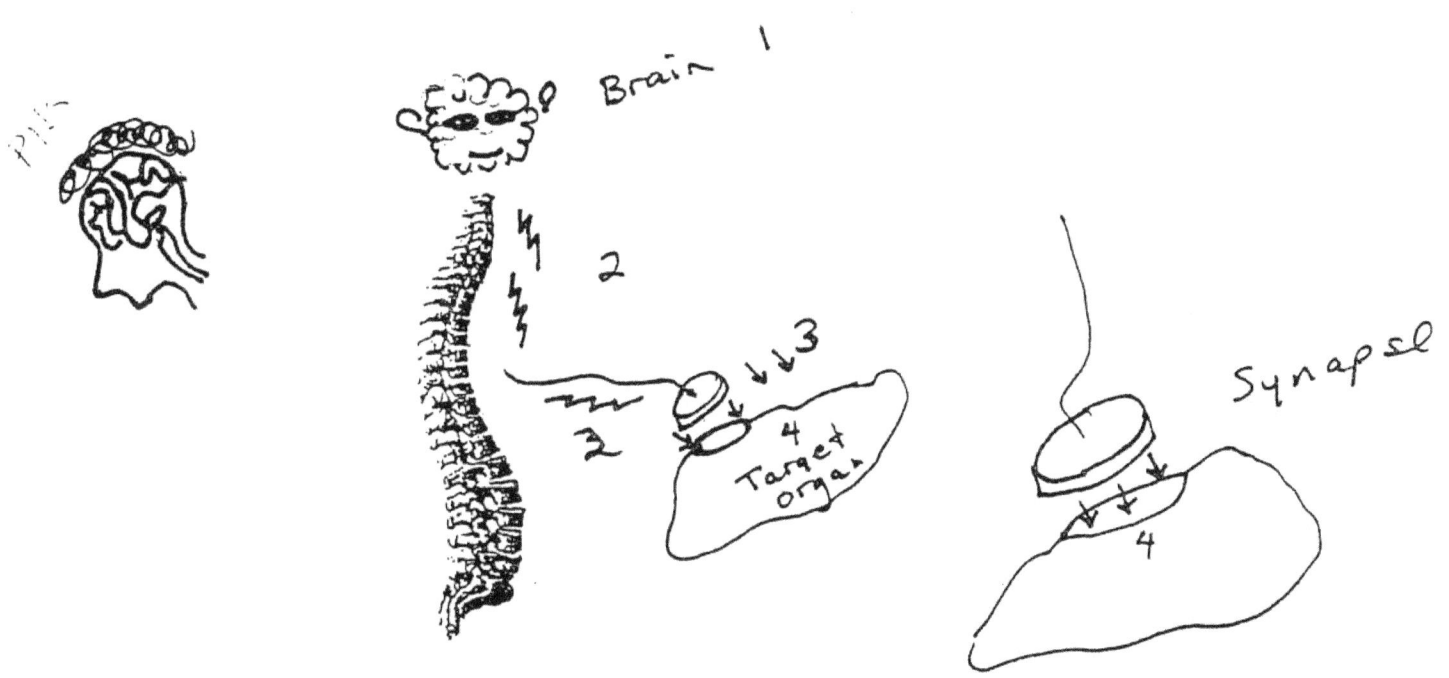

The targeted organs respond in many ways. The heart beats faster and with greater force. The lungs bronchodilate to give the body more oxygen. The kidneys constrict to shunt blood away and redirect it to more vital organs and maintain volume in the case of an injury and blood loss. The arterioles of the skeletal muscles dilate to improve circulation in the arms and legs.

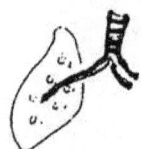

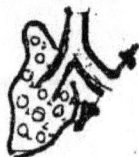

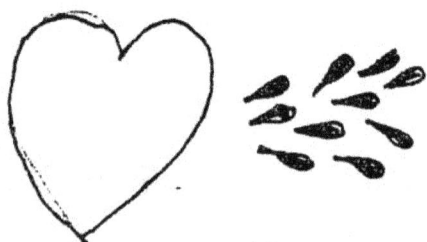

BACK-UP SYSTEM – the endocrine response

The fight or flight mechanism does all of the above very quickly – within seconds. But it can't sustain that nervous impulse for too long. To maintain that high energy level, the sympathetic nervous system activates the adrenal medula. These are two endocrine glands that sit on the top of each kidney.

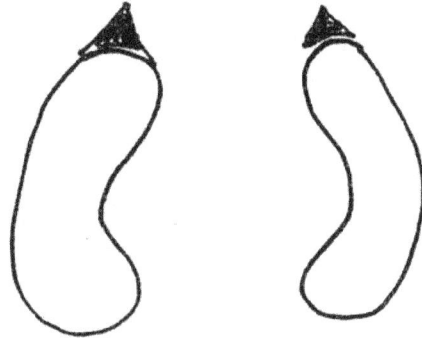

The adrenal medulae (that's the pleural of medula) secrete two neurotransmitters, epinepherine and norepinepherine. It is 80% epinepherine and 20% norepinepherine. You may remember that norepinepherine is the neurotransmitter from the sympathetic nervous system. You have probably heard of epinepherine (or adrenaline). In a cardiac arrest code blue cardiac, you will likely hear some one (not the patient) yelling "epi". It is a very potent cardiac stimulator.

The blood carries these neurotransmitters to the same sites where the sympathetic nerves were releasing norepinepherine to activate the same target organs.

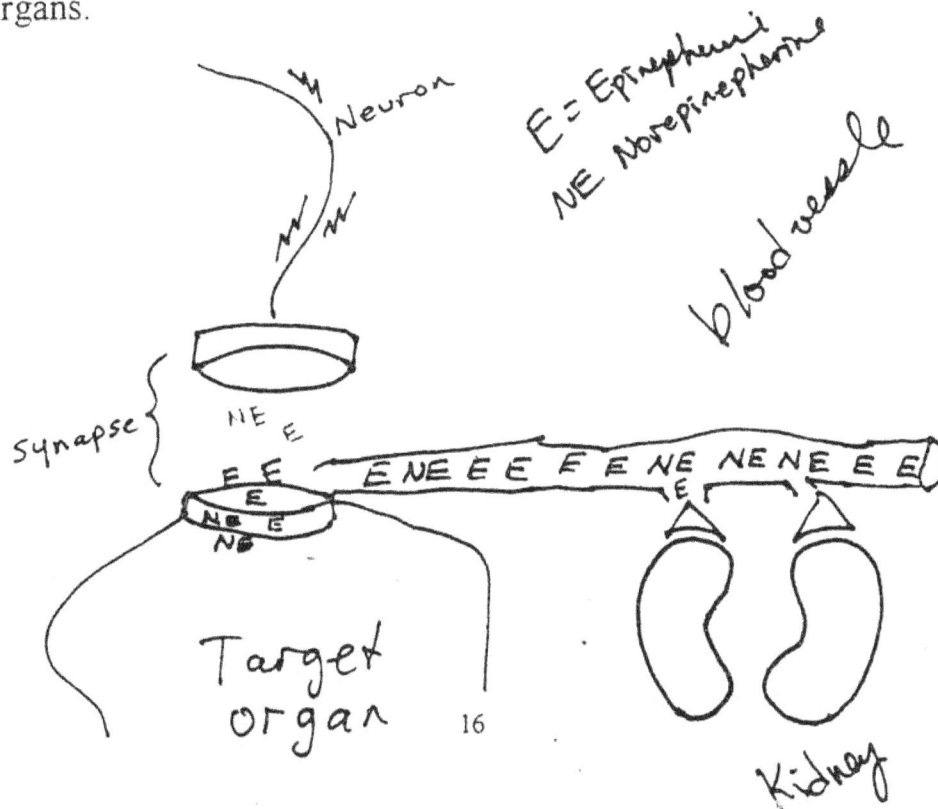

ALPHA and BETA RECEPTORS
(I did hear that term somewhere, but its Greek to me.)

Fact #1 The receptors (which we just talked about) on all the different target organs are not all alike. To be exact there are five (5) different kinds: alpha 1, alpha2, beta 1, beta 2, and dopaminergic.

Fact #2 The five different type receptors cluster on certain organs and generally promote increased activity(fight or flight) of that organ. Lets see where the different receptors are.

Alpha 1

Alpha 1 receptors are primarily located in the periferal capillaries of the skin. Stimulation of the alpha 1 receptors causes vasoconstriction of capillaries in the skin. This redirects blood flow to essential organs. Have you ever heard of a "cold fear"? The alpha 1 receptors also clamp down on arterioles in the kidney. This maintains blood pressure by retaining fluids.

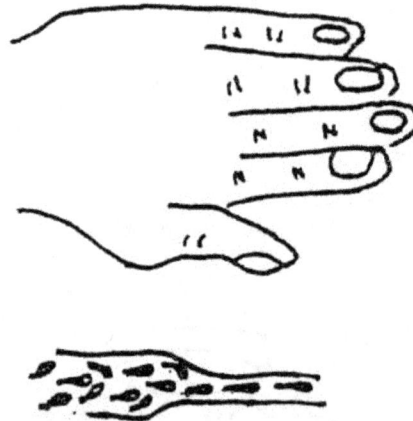

Alpha 2

Alpha 2 receptors are in the brain. Stimulating them causes vasodilation.

Beta 1

Beta 1 receptors are located primarily on the heart. Stimulation of these receptors causes increased contractility. That results in increased cardiac output. More blood flow is obviously good in those situations.

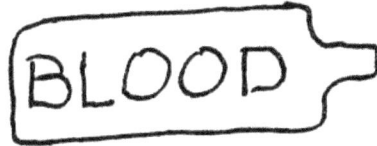

There are beta 1 receptors on the S.A. (sinoatrial) node. The S.A. node fires the electrical impulse that normally starts each heart beat. It normally fires the electrical impulse at a regular rate of 60 to 90 times a minute. That shows up as the P wave on an EKG.

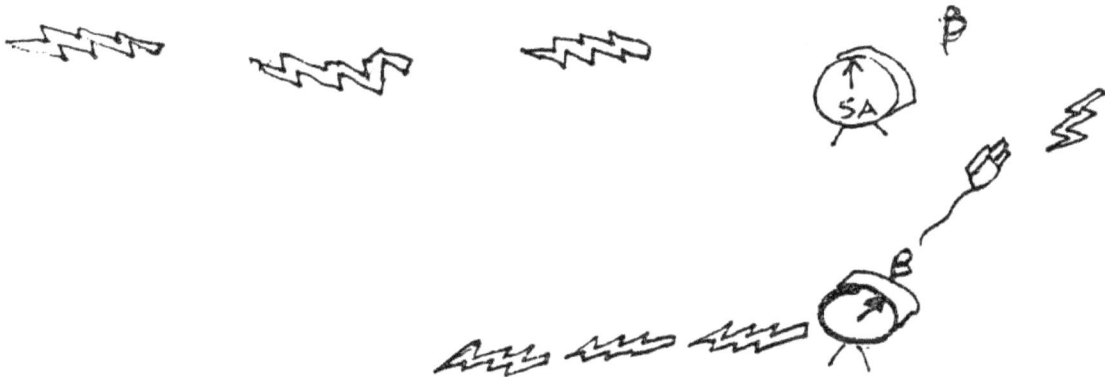

A fight or flight impulse from the sympathetic nervous system adjusts the rate to provide more blood when needed.

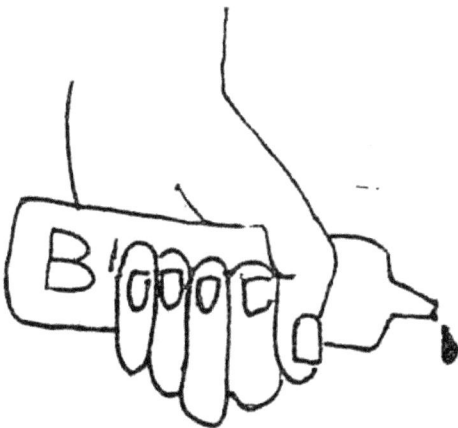

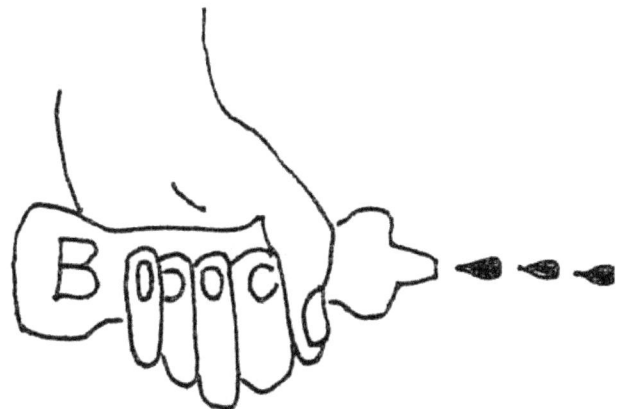

Similarly a parasympathetic impulse makes the S.A. node fire slower

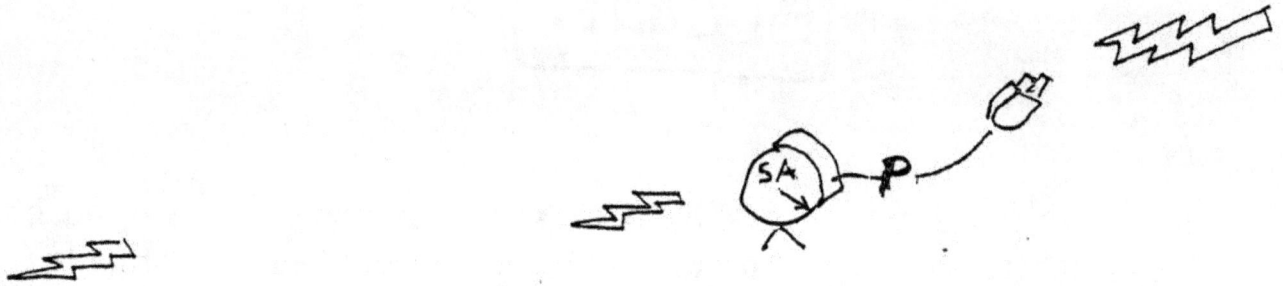

Beta 2

Beta 2 receptors are in skeletal muscles and the lungs. Excitation of beta 2 receptors causes vasodilation of blood vessels in skeletal muscles. That obviously enables a person to run faster or throw a spear. Excitation of beta 2 receptors are in the lungs cause the bronchioles to dilate and get more oxygen to the blood.

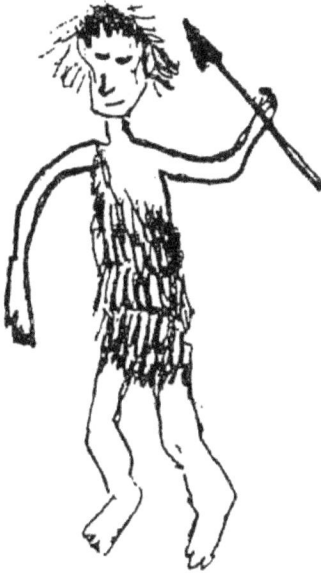

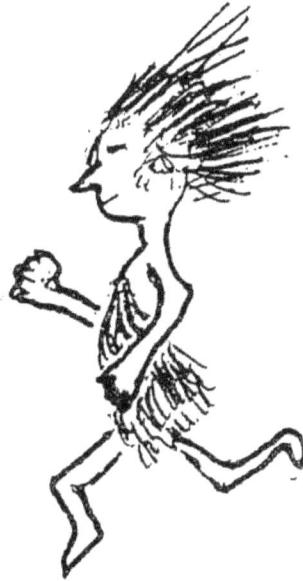

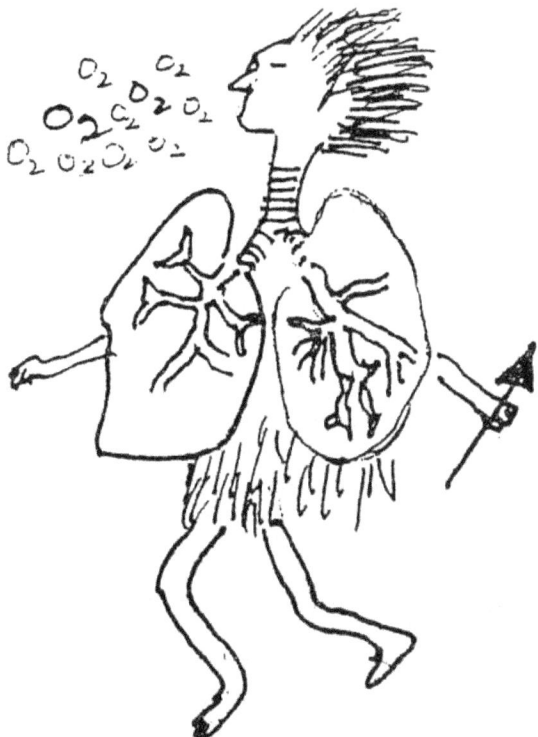

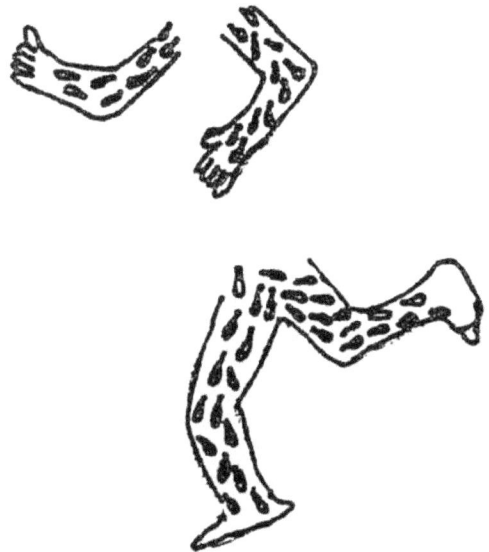

DOPAMINERGIC RECEPTORS

Dopaminergic receptors are located in the kidney and the heart (similar to beta 1). So stimulating the dopaminergic receptors increases cardiac output and urination. The increase in urine output is accomplished by dilating the renal arterioles allowing more blood flow to the kidneys.

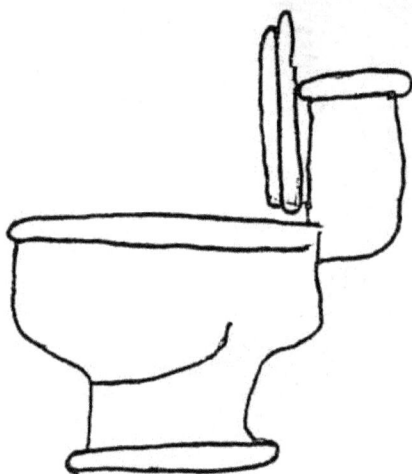

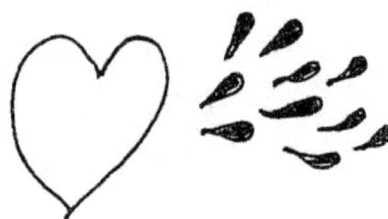

We will first look at epinepherine, norepinepherine , isuprel and dopamine and see how they work.

Epinepherine

Epinepherine is secreted by the adrenal medullae directly into the bloodstream, or it can be withdrawn from a one ml. vial and injected via a syringe. Epinepherine is the strongest and most encompasing adrenergic stimulent (or agonist). It stimulates alpha 1, beta 1 and beta 2 receptors. It stimulates alpha 1 receptors and constricts arterioles in the skin. That redistributes blood to the brain and skeletal muscles. The beta 1 property is a strong cardiac stimulent. It increases the heart rate and strength of contraction or overall cardiac output. The beta 2 properties cause powerful bronchodilation. The general purpose is great oxygen demands in fight or flight situations. That demands bronchodilation.

Lets look at using epinepherine in anaphylactic shock caused by a severe asthmatic reaction. That would be characterized by near suffocating from bronchoconstriction and severe hypotension from widespread vasodilation, and swelling of the glottis (wind pipe).

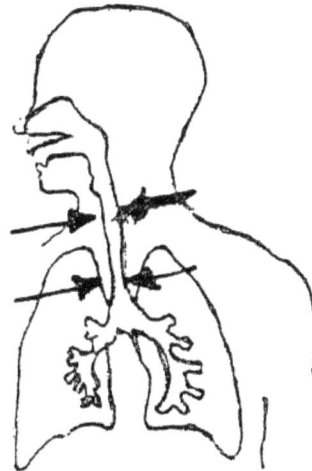

By stimulating alpha 1 receptors and constricting the peripheral arterioles blood pressure is increased and blood flow redirected to vital organs.

"Shock shock shock....epi....shock shock shock...epi"

Lets also look at epinepherine in code blue situations. Epinepherine via its beta 1 receptor effect stimulates the heart to beat faster and more forcefully which reverses cardiac standstill as well as hypotension. By its alpha effects epinephrine causes generalized arteriolar vasoconstriction which helps to maintain an adequate blood pressure. Maintaining an adequate blood pressure is critical. It keeps an adequate blood flow to the brain heart and kidneys. Its beta 2 effect tends to counteract bronchoconstriction which often accompanies the "code blue" state. Epinepherine or "epi" is the first drug in cardiac arrest. Do you remember "Shock, shock, shock, epi, shock, shock, shock..."? We will get into this later. Here the epi is restarting the sinus node after the defibrillation has stopped all ectopic electrical activity. We explain defibrillation in the conduction section.

DOPAMINE AND DOPAMINERGIC RECEPTORS

There is a fifth kind of receptor (in addition to alpha and beta) called dopaminergic receptors. They respond to dopamine. (duh) They are mostly in the kidneys and the heart. Dopaminergic stimulation of the kidneys will cause dilation of renal blood vessels. This causes more blood flow through the kidneys and as a result more urination. That's why low doses (up to 5 mics/kg/min) are called renal doses of dopamine. At this point it has little effect on the heart and peripheral circulation.

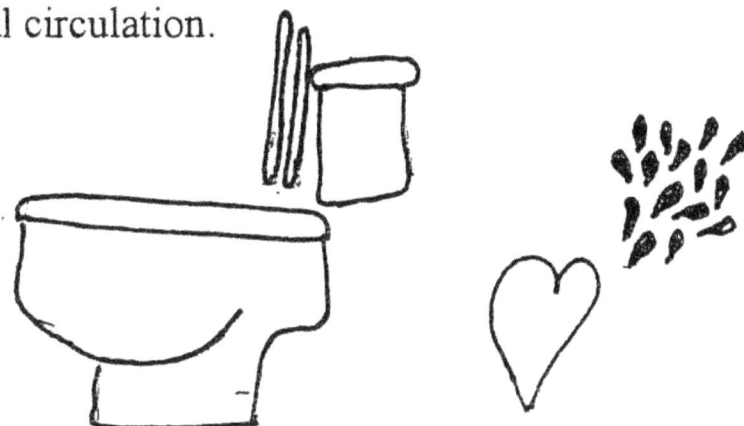

Stimulation of dopaminergic receptors (by I.V. dopamine at 5 mics/kg/min) will increase heart rate like beta 1 stimulation. Dopamine also stimulates beta 1 receptors. So for treatment of shock dopamine is generally the first choice. It causes increased heart rate and increased force of contraction – or increased cardiac output. But the reason it's the #1 choice of I.C.U nurses is that it reduces the risk of renal failure.

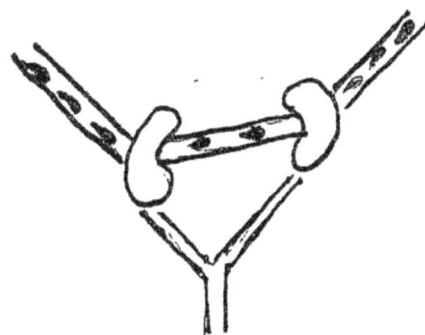

In high doses (>20 mics/kg/min) dopamine stimulates alpha receptors which then counteract the dopamine receptors in the kidney. Then it starts to act more like norepinepherine. (Do you remember constricting peripheral vasculature and renal arteries to direct blood to vital organs)

NOREPINEPHERINE or LEVOPHED
(Levophed is also called leave em dead)

Norepineiperine, the stimulent we know so well, is synthetically produced as a drug we know as levophed. In ICU situations levophed is generally hung after dopamine. The primary benefit is to cause peripheral vasoconstriction. Dopamine is much more effective at speeding up the heart. Norepinepherine has both Beta 1 and Beta 2 effects. Epinepherine has stronger Beta effects. Norepinepherine has much stronger Alpha effects. It is used for profound hypotension after dopamine has failed to raise the blood pressure. One of the problems with levophed is that the vasoconstriction may be too strong. The heart can't pump against so much resistance (afterload) and causes less perfusion overall. Levophed is most useful in cases of circulatory collapse. The best example of that is septic shock.

DOBUTREX or DOBUTAMINE

Dobutrex is primarily a beta 1 stimulent. It mainly stimulates the heart to beat more forcefully. It does not significantly increase heart rate. In congestive heart failure, that feature increases cardiac output without increasing oxygen demands. That is the major advantage over other cardiac stimulants.

Dobutamine is similar to dopamine. Dobutrex has less Alpha and more Beta 1 effect than dopamine. This is therefore is a good drug in situations where cardiac output (like post MI or CHF), not hypotension (septic shock) is the predominant problem. Similar to dopamine dobutrex preserves or enhances renal blood flow (and as a result urination).

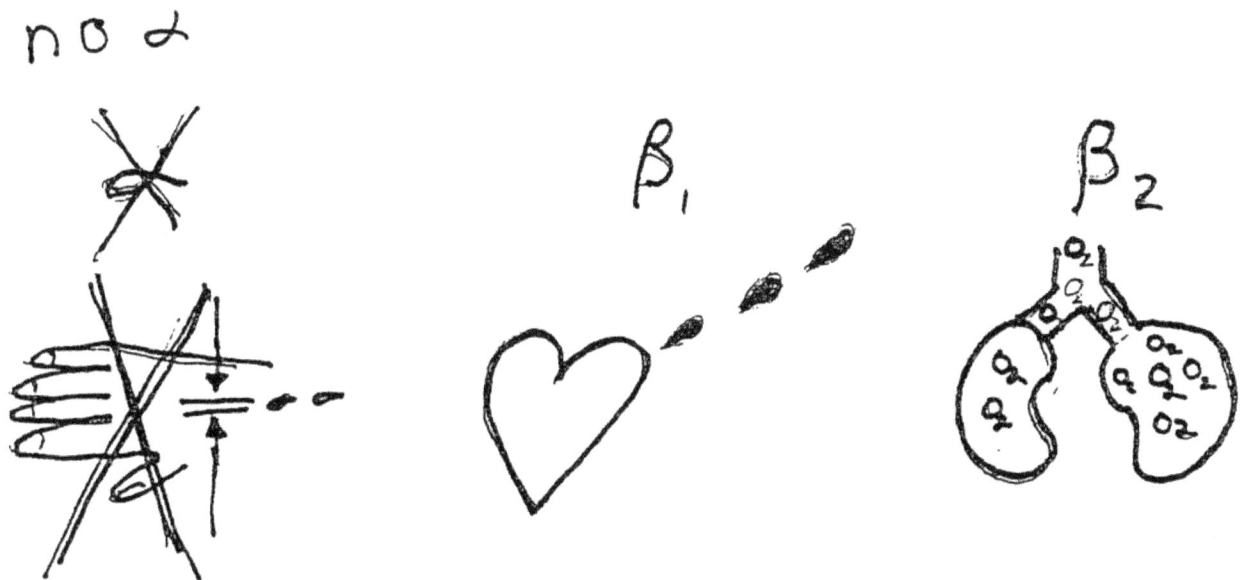

ISOPROTERINOL or ISUPREL

Isuprel is a beta stimulant. Isuprel acts only on beta 1 and beta 2. It was the first drug to affect only beta receptors (a little medical history).

Via its beta 1 action it can restart the heart following cardiac arrest. It can increase cardiac output during shock. It can overcome A.V. block. It increases cardiac output (beta 1). It dilates peripheral arterioles. (beta 2 effects)

As the beta 2 agonist (remember that means stimulant), Isuprel decreases airway resistance in patients with severe life threatening asthma. However more recently beta 2 selective drugs (that act only on beta 2) have come along. So Isuprel is no longer used as a first line drug for bronchoconstriction.

NEOSYNEPHERINE Pure Alpha stimulation

You probably know of neosynepherine as nose drops for nasal congestion. By vasoconstricting the capillaries it is opening the air passages. Capillaries in the nasal passages are a good example of peripheral vessels that areclosed by alpha stimulation. Neosynepherine is available I.V. for profound hypotension.

AMRINONE and MILRINONE

There is a new class of inotropic agents, phosphodiesterase inhibitors. They are not alpha or beta stimulents. That means they don't stimulate electrical activity as a means of strengthening muscle contraction muscle contraction. They hold calcium in the cells. We know what that means: stronger contractions. They are only available I.V.

A few new drugs, Proamitine and Natrecor

I ran across a new drug the other day, midodrine (proamitine). I had never heard of it. It turns out to be an alpha 1 stimulent used for orthostatic hypotension, That makes sence.By stimulation of the the alpha 1 receptors, the peripheral vasculature contracts. That forces blood to other parts like the head.

Another new drug is Natrecor. Similar to all the alpha and beta blockers and stimulants (which comprise most of this book), natrecor is a medication that adds to a "natural medication." In this case it adds BNP (brain-type naturatic peptide). Huh?

What's that? In response to excessive stretch, the heart produces two things. When the atria are overstretched, the atria produce atrial naturetic peptide (ANP). When the ventricles are overstretched they produce brain type naturetic peptide. If you are interested a peptide is a protein hormone (chain of amino acids). These two peptides act to reduce after load of the heart. They do this in two ways. As a vasodilator theydilate both veins and arteries. And they diurese the body of salt and water to reduce the volume of blood. Of these two BNP is much stronger.

Heart failure can be diagnosed by measuring BNP levels in the blood. Less than 100 is a normal heart. 100 to 1000 can mean heart failure and greater than 1000 means the heart is being stretched too much – which is a sign of heart failure. We don't measure ANP.

For therapeutic intervention of congestive heart failure we give high doses of BNP (Natrecor). They are much higher than the body produces on its own.

BLOCKERS

All of the fight or flight stimulation we just learned about can be reversed. A blocker stops the norepinepherine from reaching the alpha and beta receptors we just talked about. A blocker impedes the neurotransmitter at the receptor site

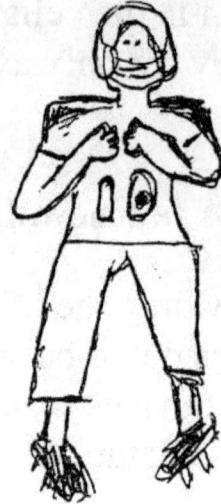

ALPHA BLOCKERS

Lets look at alpha 1 blockers. (or antagonists) Off the top of your head, what do you think they do? They block alpha 1's. They block the neurotransmitter at the alpha 1 sites. Where are the alpha 1 sites? On smooth muscle. Duh!,. Stimulating alpha 1 sites contracts smooth muscle. Blocking alpha 1 receptors dilates smooth muscles. That lowers blood pressure – which is usually the purpose.

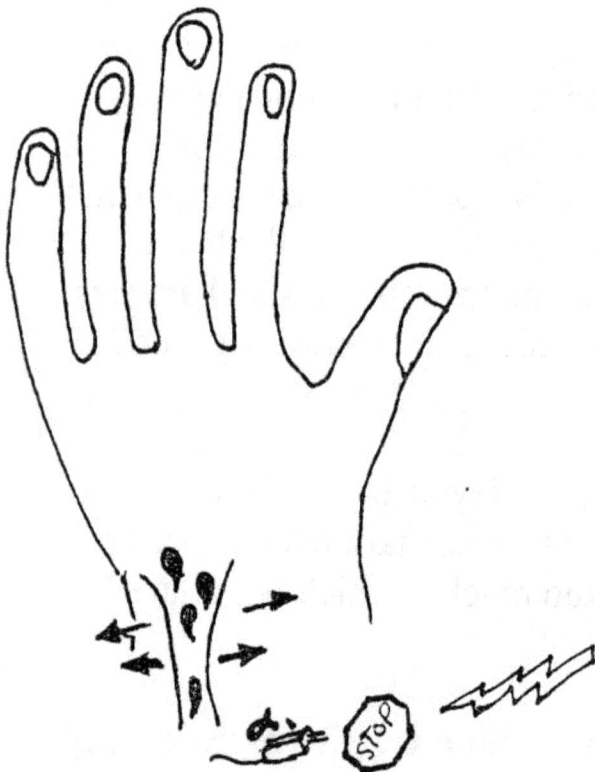

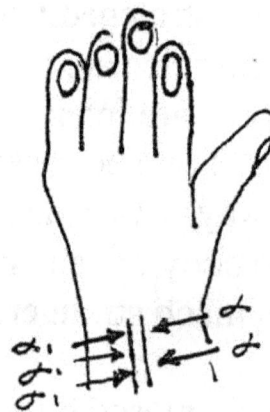

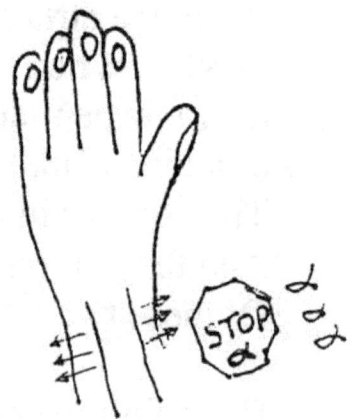

30

Prazosin (Minipress) and terazoson (Hytrin) and cardura decrease peripheral vascular resistance and lower arterial blood pressure by causing the relaxation of both arterial and venous smooth muscle. These drugs cause only minimal changes in cardiac out put and renal blood flow. Minipress and Hytrin are commonly used for benign prostatic hypertrophy since they also cause relaxation of the bladder sphincter.

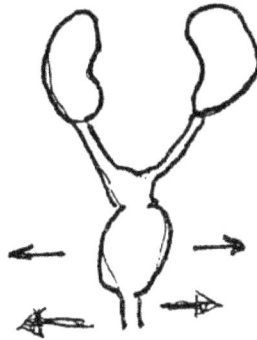

What if an I.V. dopamine or epinepherine infusion infiltrates? Their powerful alpha 1 vasoconstrictive quality would impede the local blood flow to the point of starving the tissues, or necrosis. The answer? Give Regitine subcutaneous. This alpha 1 antagonist blocks the alpha 1 agonist at the site of infiltration and allows arteriolar vasodilation and perfusion of the tissues.

ALPHA 2 STIMULENTS

Clonadine (Catapress) and methyldopa are alpha 2 stimulents. They are very potent vasodilators. Alpha 2 receptors are in the brain. Catapress patches are used to stop nicotine addiction.

BETA BLOCKERS
(I've heard that term. What does it mean?)

Beta blockers block beta 1 and beta 2 receptors. They do this by attaching themselves to the receptor and preventing the neurotransmittor from reaching the target organ. Lets look at Inderal (propanolol). Inderal blocks beta 1 and beta 2. So it would reduce cardiac output by decreasing heart rate and contratility (beta 1) and it will block natural bronchodilation which we call bronchoconstriction or choking.

That's blocking beta 2. That is the most dangerous possible side effect of Indreral. In a patient with C.O.P.D. or asthma this could be fatal.

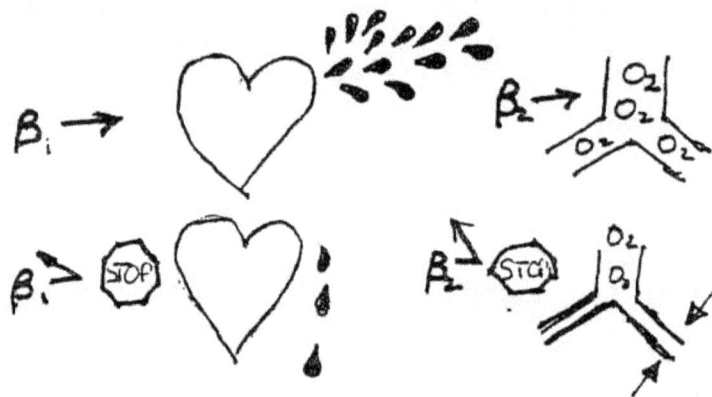

There is a new word to learn: **NONSELECTIVE**. Nonselective means that the Inderal does not select the beta receptor it attaches to. It attaches to both beta 1 and beta 2 . This is important because our next class of beta blockers are selective.

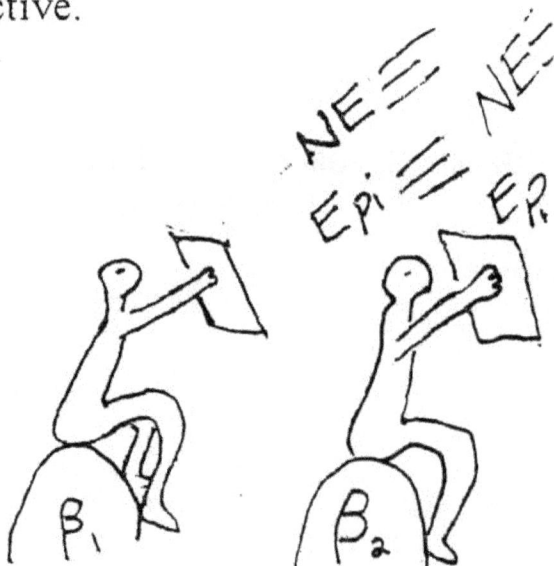

SELECTIVE BETA BLOCKERS

Drugs that block only beta 1 receptors are called selective beta blockers. Drugs that block only beta 1 receptors slow down the heart without unwanted bronchoconstriction.

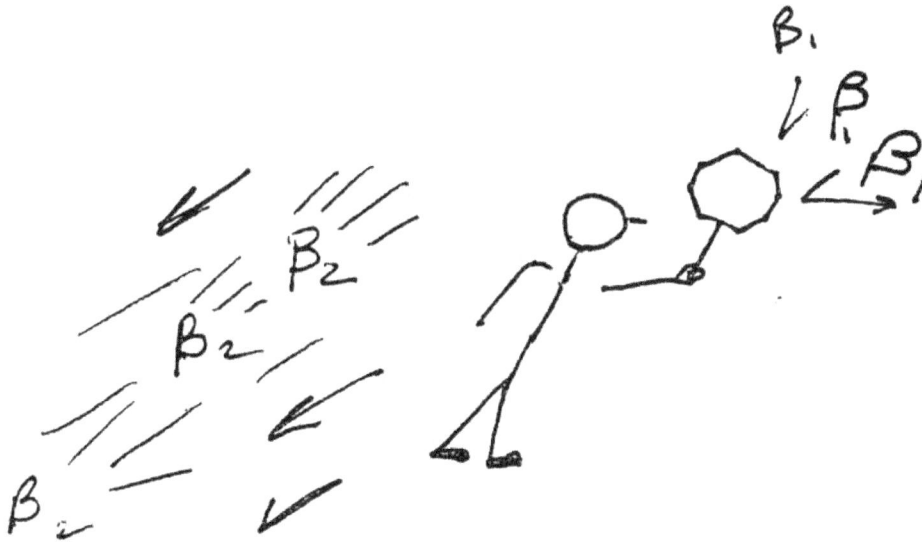

Metopropolol (Lopresser) and atenolol (Tenormin) are the most popular. They reduce heart rate, reduce force of contraction and reduce conduction of impulses through the A.V. node. They do not cause bronchoconstriction unless you use higher doses.

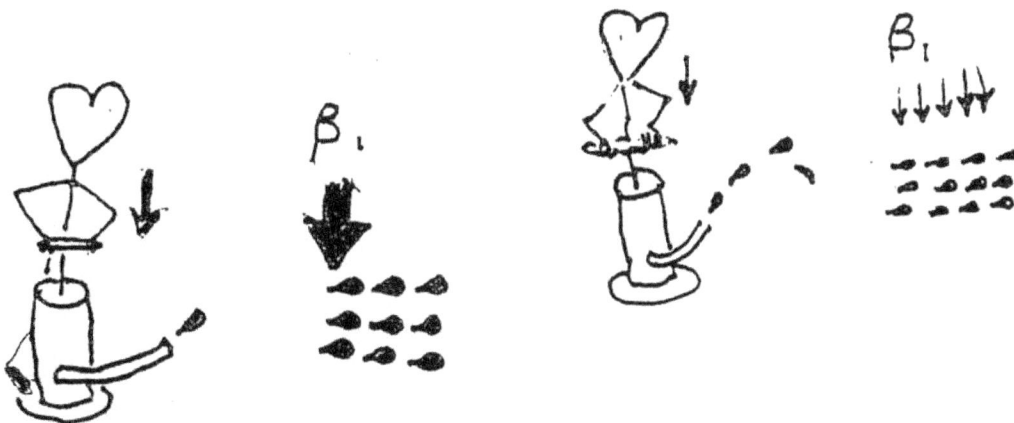

CALCIUM CHANNEL BLOCKERS

We will start with a very quick review of muscular contractions. Do not rely on it to pass cardiology boards. When the myocin and actin fibers interdigitate (Remember?) they need lots of calcium. Most of the drugs we looked at earlier get more calcium to the myocin and actin one way or another.

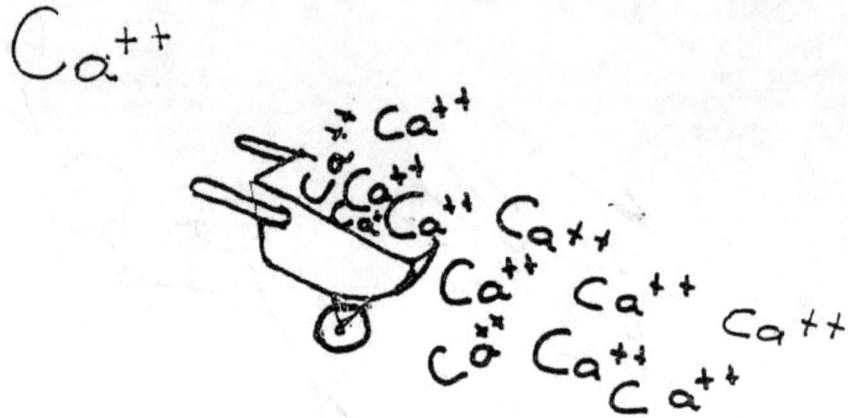

To get to the interior of each cell it flows through a channel or door. Blocking that channel (closing the door or keeping it just slightly ajar)

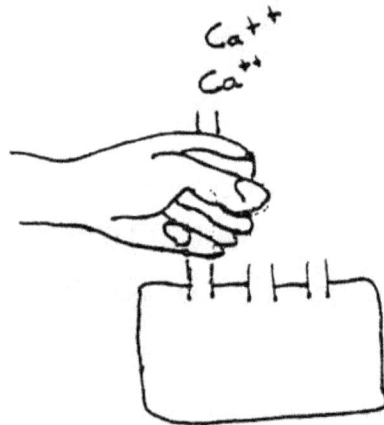

reduces the calcium, and reduces the force and velocity of contraction.

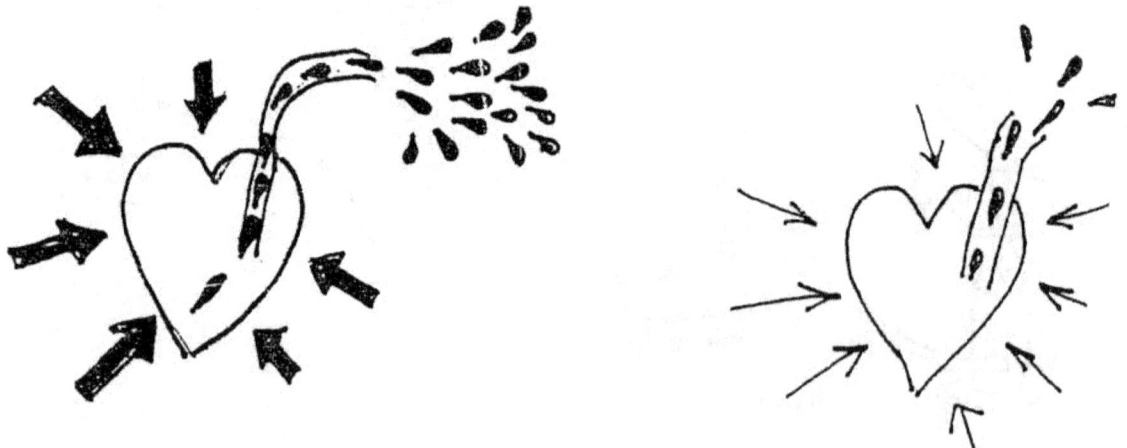

Getting away from tiny cells and looking at the Big Cardiac Picture, blocking calcium does three things. It affects angina, arrhythmias, and hypertension.

#1 Vascular smooth muscle. The smooth muscles surrounding arteries, arterioles and veins are highly dependent on changes in calcium. Remember more calcium causes the muscles around the veins to contract. That raises blood pressure. Less calcium opens vasculature or lowers blood pressure.

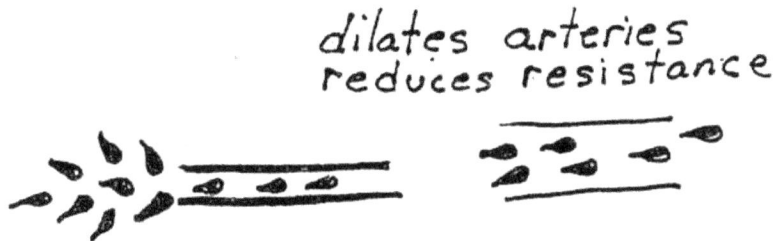

#2 Cardiac muscles. In the heart's contraction calcium is essential. More calcium means a stronger, faster contraction. If the calcium channels are blocked, cardiac contraction is slower and weaker.

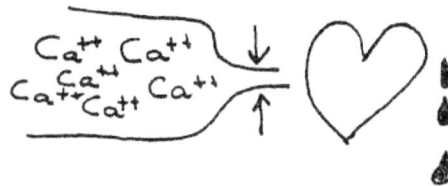

#3 Conductivity. The last step in the muscular contraction series of events is the transmission of the impulse.

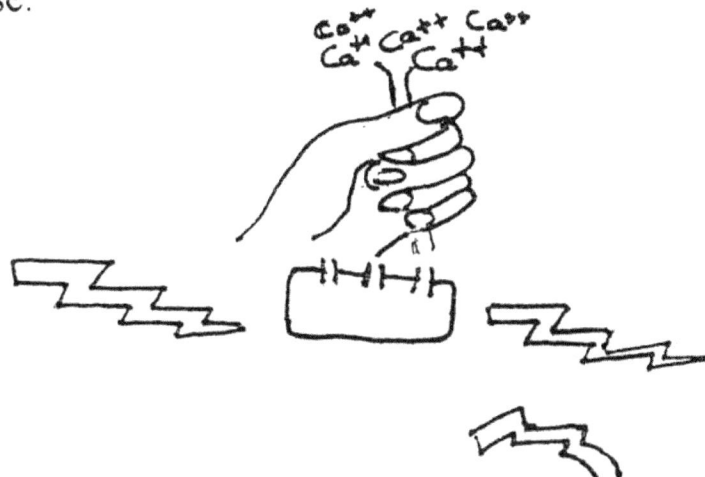

Restricting calcium slows down that series of events. That slows down the transmission of the impulse.

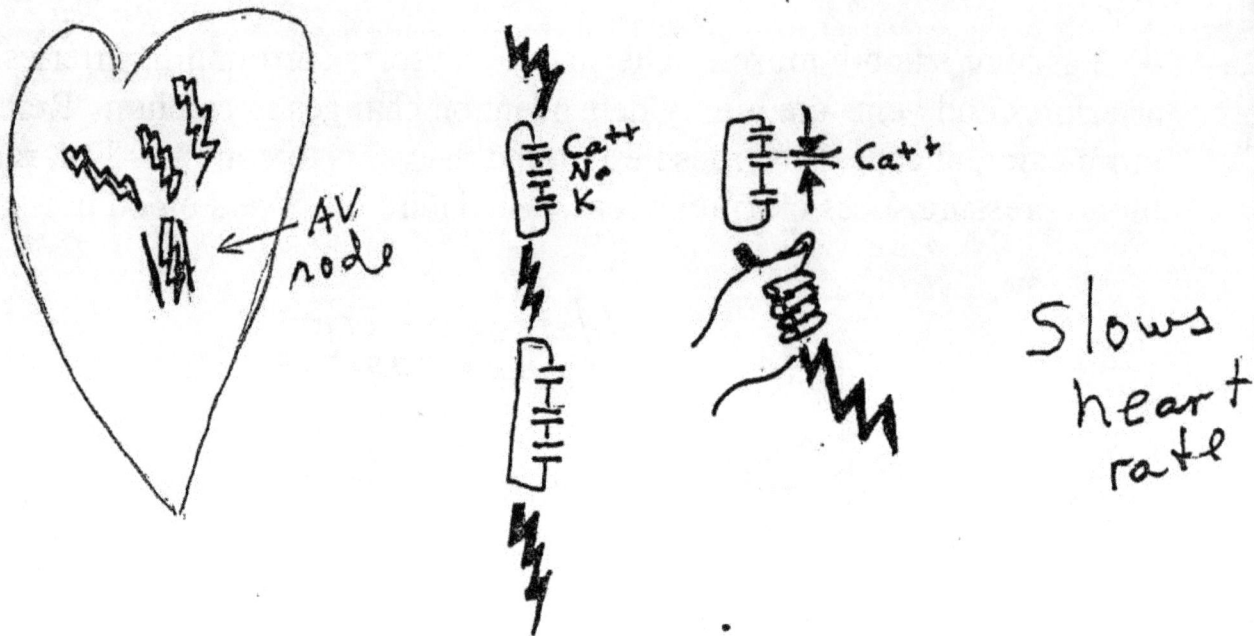

Verapamil tends to have all three effects:
It slows heart rate.
It lowers blood pressure.
It dilates coronary arteries.
That makes it a good drug for hypertension, unstable angina and SVT

Procardia or Norvasc have little effect on contractility and conduction. They work mostly on dilating vascular smooth muscles. Thus Procardia is a good drug for high blood pressure, unstable angina or vasospastic angina. It is not a good drug for supraventricular tachycardia.

BLOOD PRESSURE

You hear those words often. Typically we mean the numbers from a blood pressure cuff. You know that. Right?

Blood pressure is the oomph the heart provides to get the blood through the vasculature and back to the heart. There must be a balance between the

cardiac output

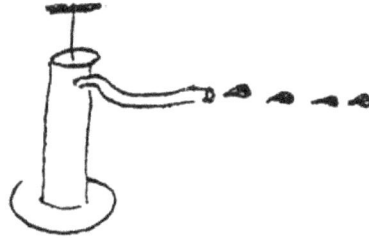

and the vascular resistance.

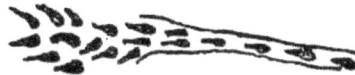

The body has two (2) systems try to keep the blood pressure within healthy limits. They are:

#1 There are pressure sensors in the aortic arch
    which activate the sympathetic nervous system.

#2 The renin–angiotensin–aldosterone system
    (the WHAT?????!!!!!!!)

RENIN-ANGIOTENSIN-ALDOSTERONE SYSTEM

When blood pressure drops the sympathetic nervous system kicks in. It signals the kidneys to release renin.

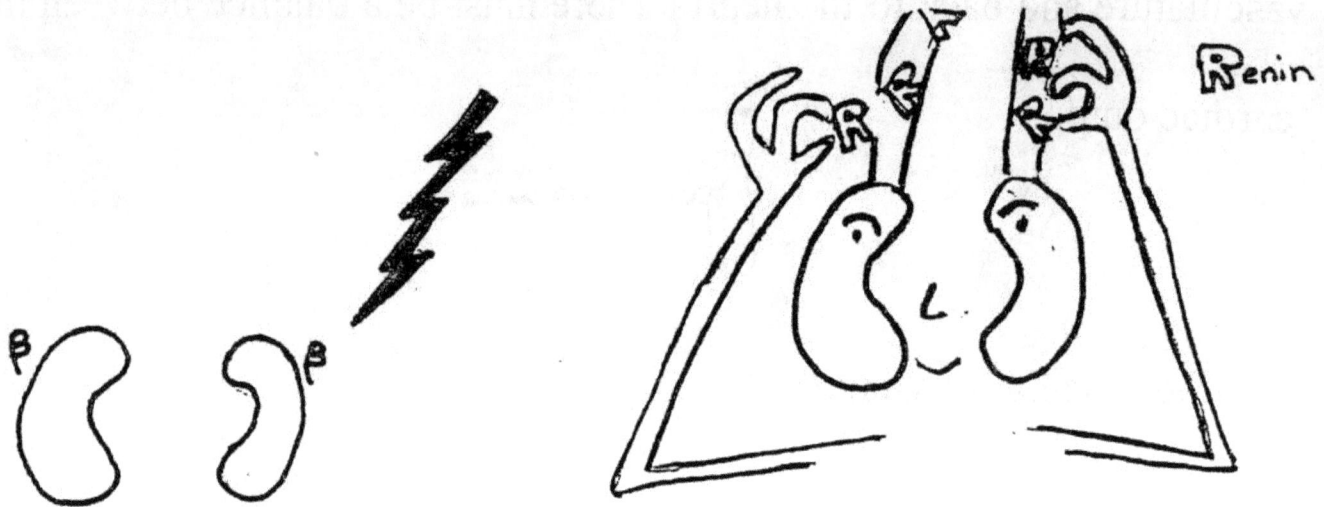

Renin converts angiotensinogen to angiotensin I. Don't worry about what that means.

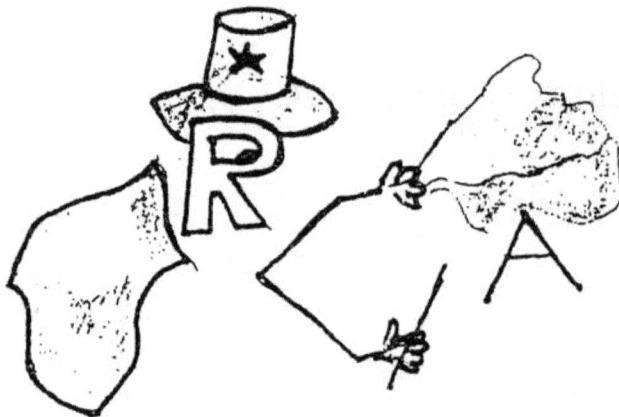

Angiotensin converting enzyme (**ACE**) converts angiotensin I to angiotensin II. One of two things you need to know is that ACE converts angiotensin I to angiotensin II.

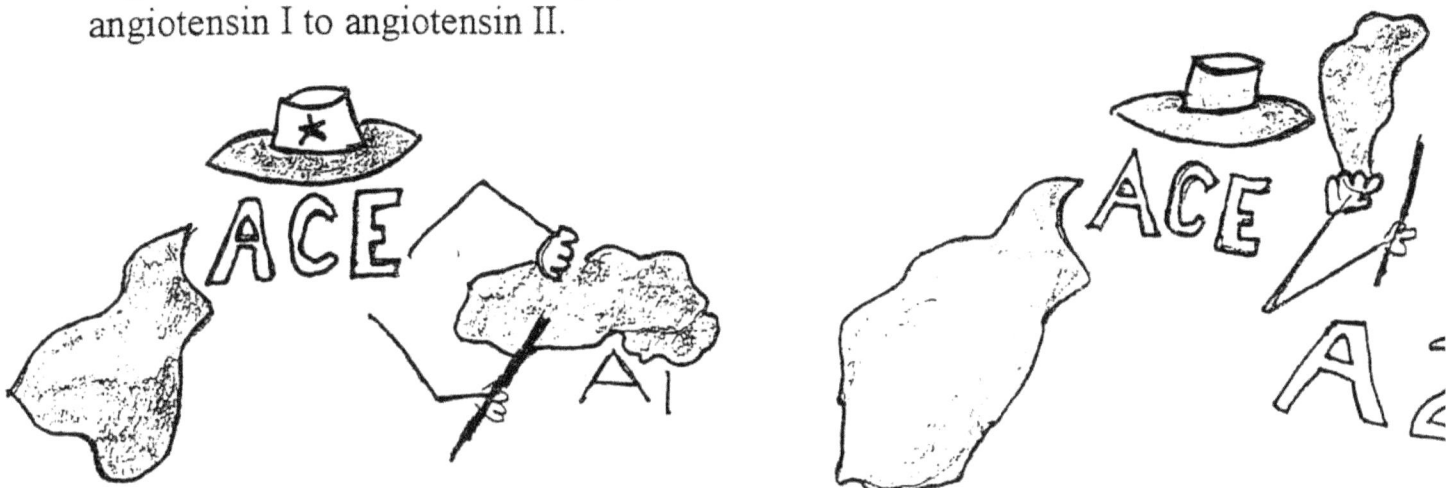

The other thing you need to know is that angiotensin II is a powerfull vasoconstrictor. That is sort of the point. Angiotensin II raises blood pressure by causing vasoconstriction. Angiotensin is 40 times more powerful than norepineherine.

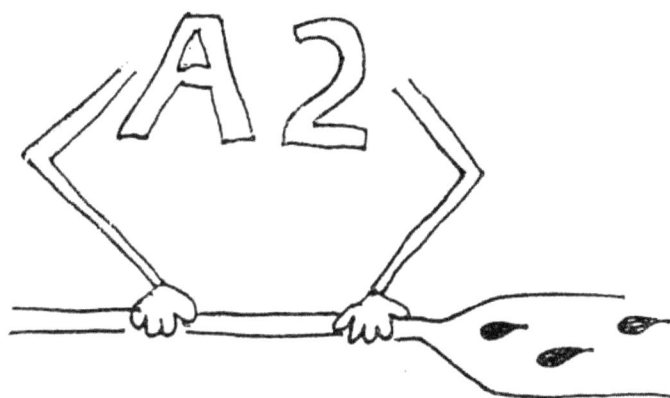

Angiotensin also stimulates the adrenal gland to secrete aldosterone.

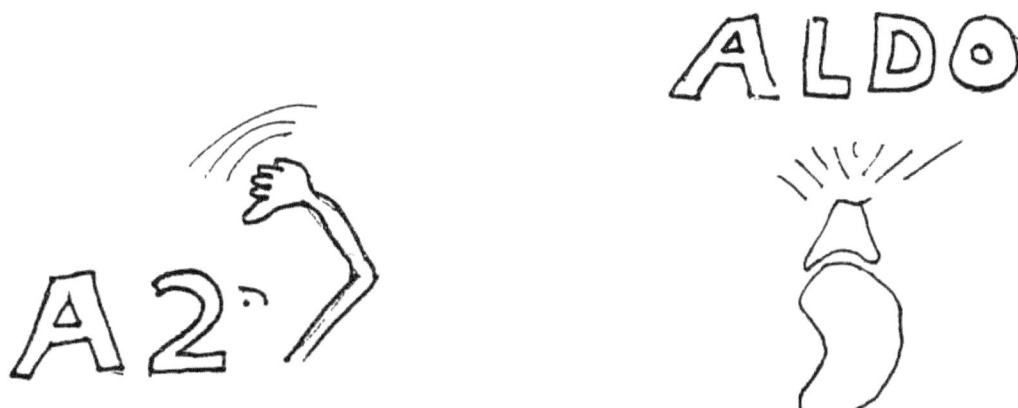

Aldosterone causes the kidneys not to excrete sodium. As you know sodium attracts water. That expands the vasculature and raises blood pressure.

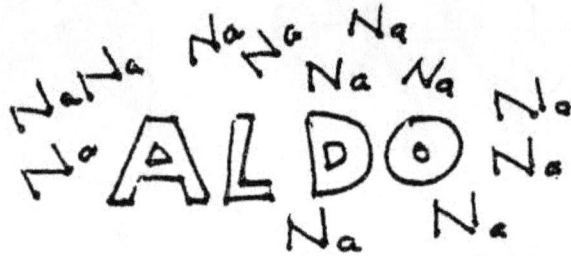

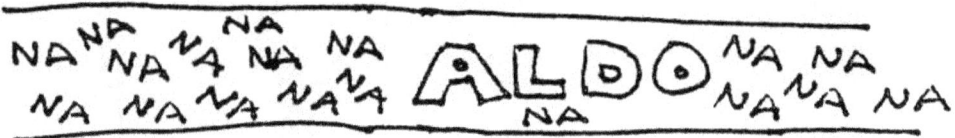

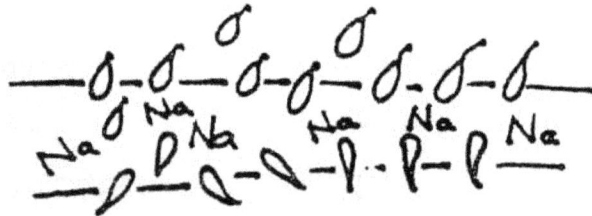

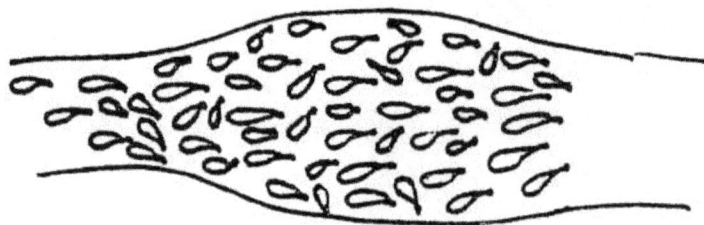

Ace Inhibitors stop the process at the point of the angiotensin converting enzyme. That prevents the vasculature from clamping down and taking in water. Or in other words, that prevents high blood pressure. Ace inhibitors lower blood pressure without affecting cardiac rate or contractility. (More on this to follow)

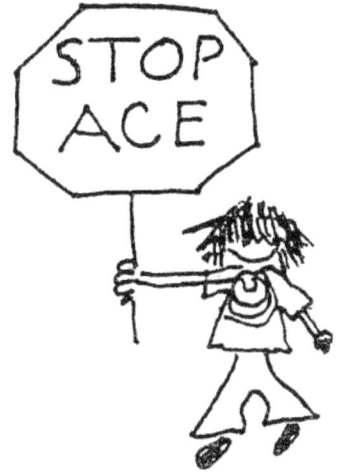

HOW THE SYMPATHETIC NERVOUS SYSTEM RAISES BLOOD PRESSURE

The sympathetic does this to protect the body by making sure enough blood gets to vital organs. What would be an example of this? Lets look at our cave man friend. He just cut his finger on a spear while trying to open a coconut.

He bleeds.

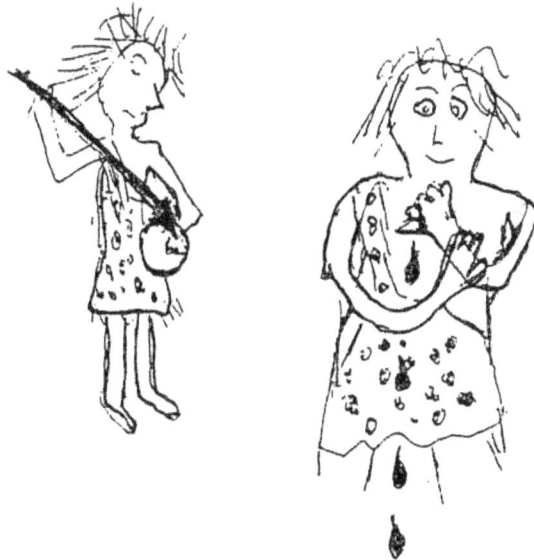

His body senses the blood loss. The body knows this from pressure sensors in the aortic arch. There is a little man whose job it is to constantly watch blood pressure.

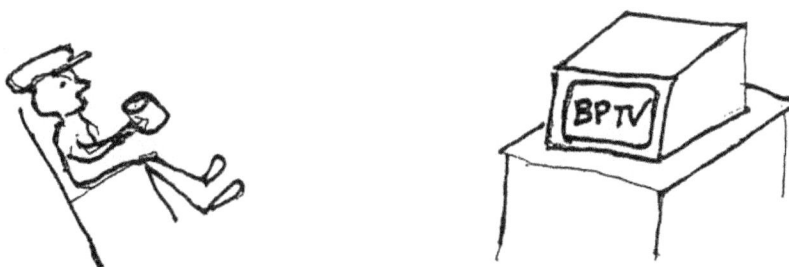

When it drops due to blood loss,

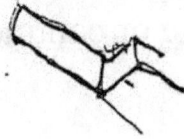

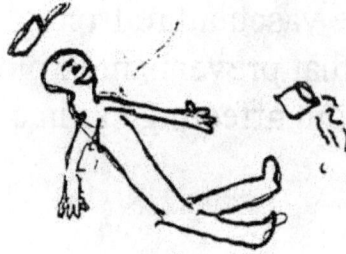

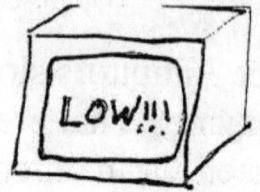

He gets on the phone and calls the sympathetic nervous system. The sympathetic nervous system wants to make sure the brain gets enough blood. So it shoots out an impulse.

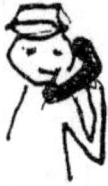

It stimulates the beta 1 receptors in the heart to beat faster and more forcefully

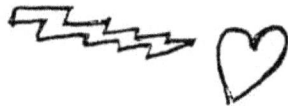

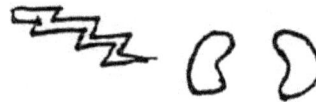

The impulse also reaches the beta 1 receptors in the kidneys. That causes the renin-angiotensin-aldosterone system to pull in more water and clamp down on the vasculature.

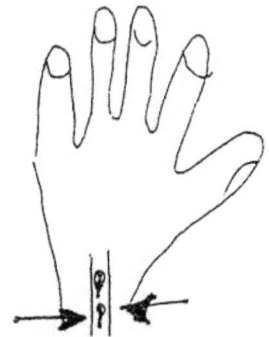

Additionally the sympathetic impulse causes the alpha 1 receptors to close down the peripheral vasculature.

All this means more fluid in less space or higher blood pressure. Higher blood pressure can be good or bad. The main point of this book is that medications are working with those blood pressure systems – either enhancing them or squelching them. Now lets go to bad high blood pressure, the kind we want to control.

HIGH BLOOD PRESSURE

High blood pressure is more blood in the arteries than they can easily carry.

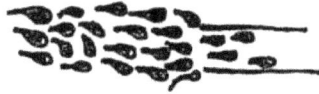

Normally to meet the body's requirements for more blood the heart pumps faster and stronger. To accommodate the increased circulation the vasculature expands elastically by decreasing the muscular tone in the small arteries.

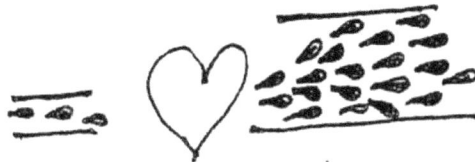

If, for whatever reason, it can't expand enough, that causes high blood pressure.

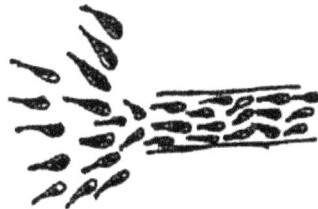

Lets first look at vascular anatomy. We can better understand high blood pressure if we know a little more about veins and arteries. All blood vessels are surrounded by layers of muscles. When they contract the the diameter of the vein or artery contracts.

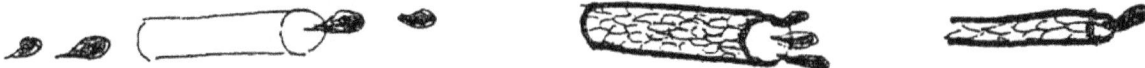

Here we see a ring of vascular smooth muscle. If they contract the diameter will get smaller. Don't forget the flow of sodium potassium and calcium as they contract (after the sympathetic nervous system stimulation).

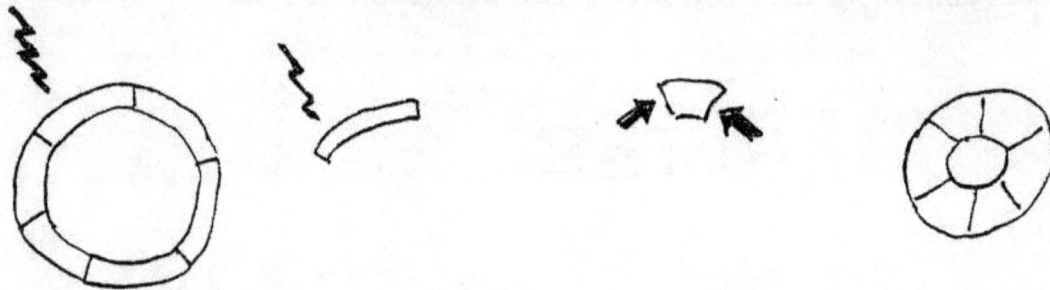

The vascular smooth muscle act a lot like cardiac muscles. They respond to sympathetic stimulation.

Under fight or flight conditions beta 1stimulation produces faster and more forceful contractions. That means more cardiac output.

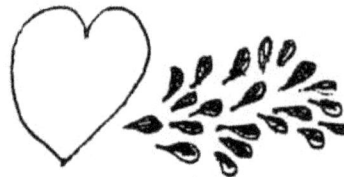

Fight or flight sympathetic stimulation of alpha 1 receptors clamps down on peripheral vasculature. So we have more blood trying to push through the narrowed vasculature.

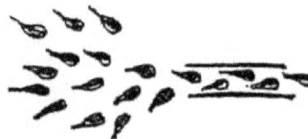

That means higher blood pressure. If the blood vessels stretch elastically, the pressure doesn't go up too much.

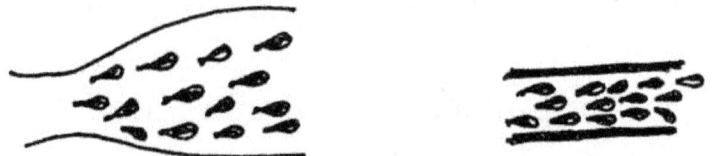

High blood pressure means the heart has to work much harder. Over a period of years that extra effort damages the heart and causes congestive heart failure. That pressure backs up to the brain where it can cause a stroke. It can damage the small arterioles in the kidneys and similarly the small blood vessels in the eyes.

BAD HIGH BLOOD PRESSURE

Most commonly high blood pressure begins with excessive salt consumption. We need about two to three grams of sodium. A Mc Donalds, Burger King, Wendy's diet (of Big Macs, Whoopers and Classics with Cheese) can easily exceed six grams of sodium.

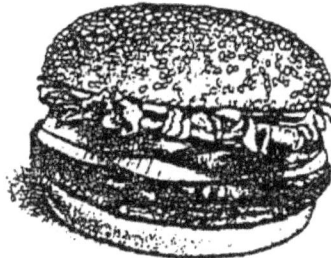

The kidneys can't excrete (micturate, urinate, pee-pee) all of the salt.

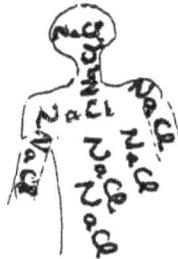

So they retain water to dilute the high sodium concentration which raises the blood pressure.

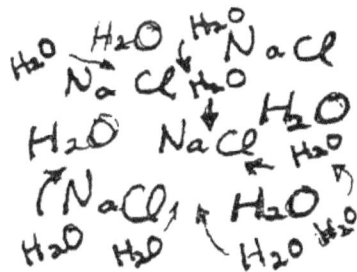

Over a period of time the continually overstretched vasculature loses its elasticity. That's called atherosclerosis or hardening of the arteries. If the veins can't stretch easily then it will be very difficult to push any extra blood through. Also the high blood pressure damages the blood vessels over time and causes further atherosclerosis and worsening of the high blood pressure problem.

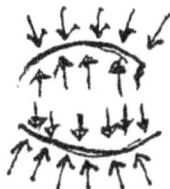

Another cause of long term hypertension is the so called Type A personality.

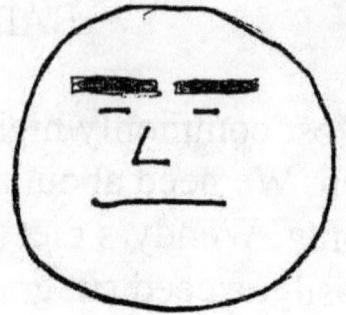

All of that constant adrenalin maintains the vasculature in a constant state of contraction.

This causes the muscle layers surrounding the arteries to lose their elasticity. Also a layer of plaque builds up. That is called arteriosclerosis.

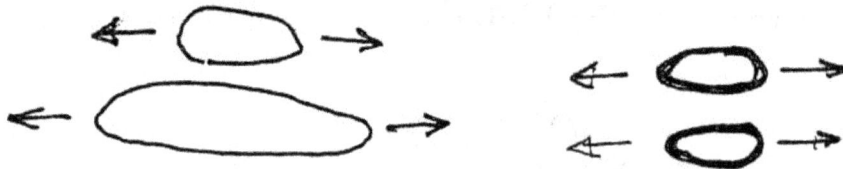

In the same way the renal arteries harden and narrow.

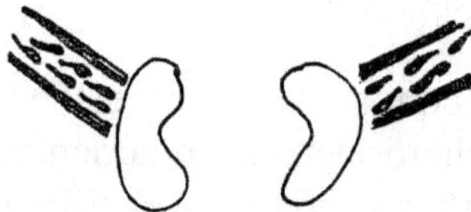

The kidneys get less blood through the hardened and narrowed renal arteries.

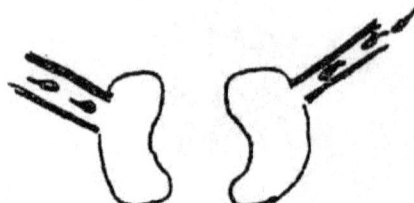

At this point the kidneys make things worse: Because of the hardened and narrowed renal arteries, there is less blood flowing through.

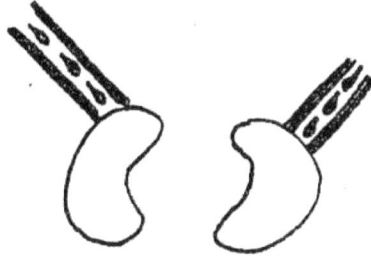

The kidneys perceive this condition as a loss blood (as in a wound)

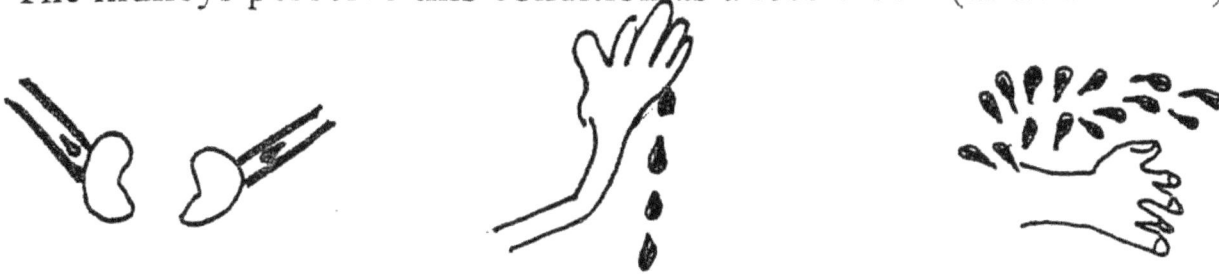

and release renin which starts the renin-angiotensin cycle. That causes the system to pull in more water and causes the vasculature to clamp down further.

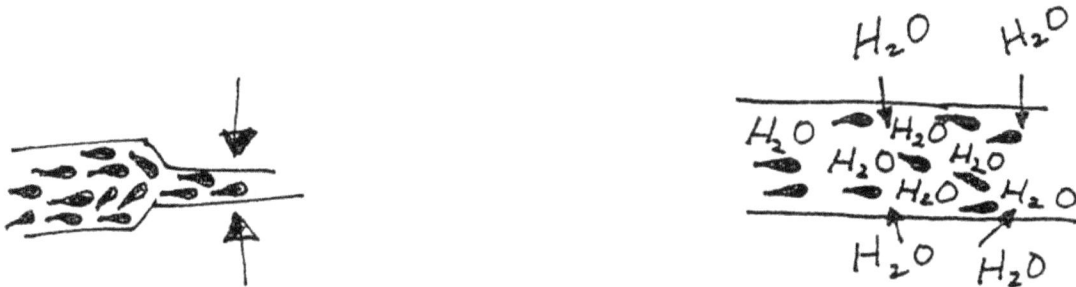

That higher blood pressure can cause a stroke, cause blindness or damage the heart. Small delicate veins in the kidneys and eyes are the most vulnerable.

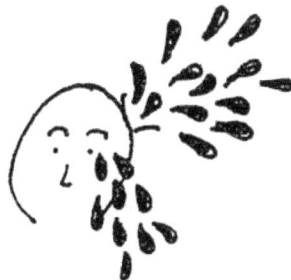

DRUGS for HYPERTENSION

To combat hypertension there are medications. To understand these medications is probably the reason you are reading this book. If there is any other reason please tell me. Roughly speaking there are four things to do.

(1) Relax with or without medication

(2) Reduce the volume with diuretics

(3) Reduce the volume of blood **pumped** by reducing the heart rate and contractility with beta blockers (not changing the volume)

(4) Open up the vasculature with alpha blockers, beta blockers or ace inhibitors

or

(5) A combination of the above

Diuretics. This seems pretty obvious. If the vasculature won't expand to allow more blood flow, then we reduce the blood volume. Taking out the water does this. There are two important points to keep in mind. One: watch the blood pressure. It might drop too much. The other frequent side effect 0f diuretics is losing potassium. Even with potassium sparing diuretics you must be aware of potassium levels and the signs and symptoms of high and low levels of potassium.

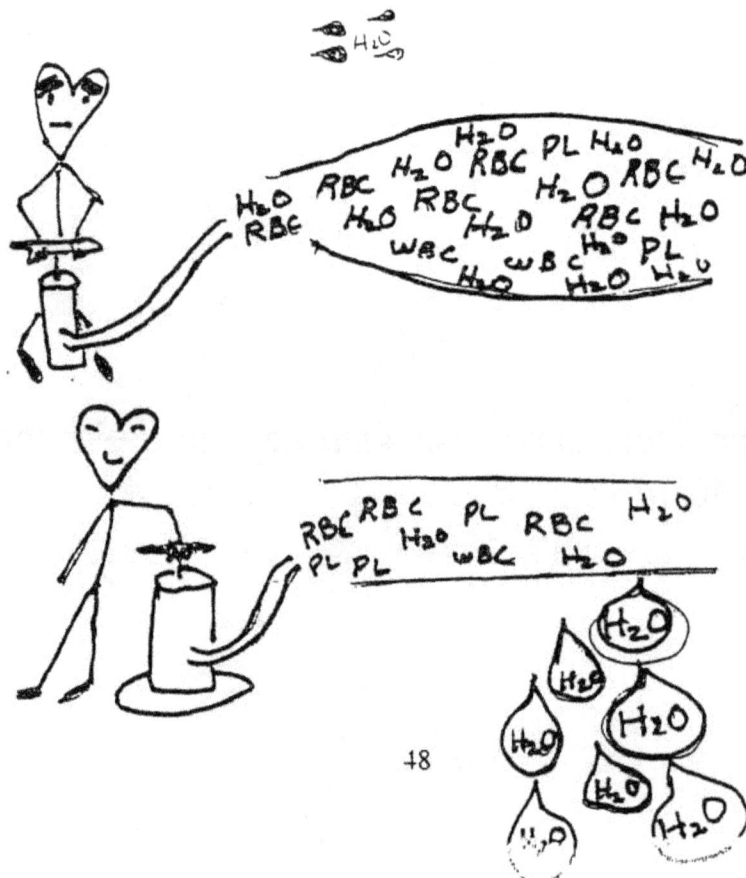

BETA BLOCKERS for HYPERTENSION (Words fail me)

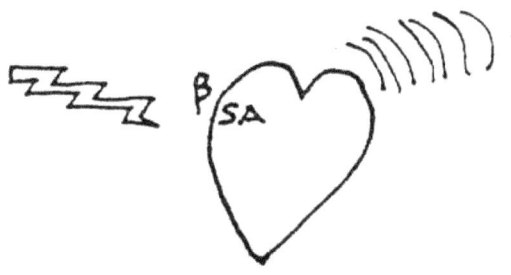

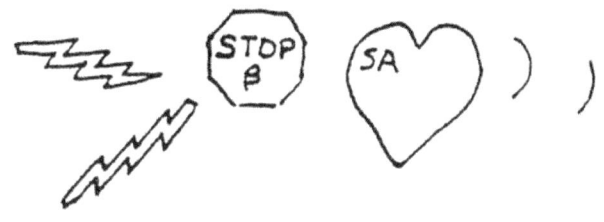

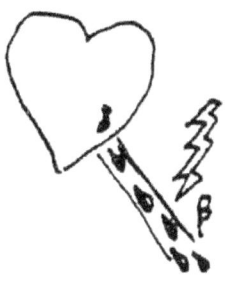

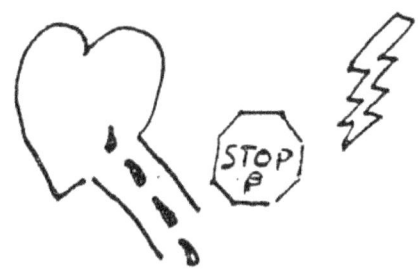

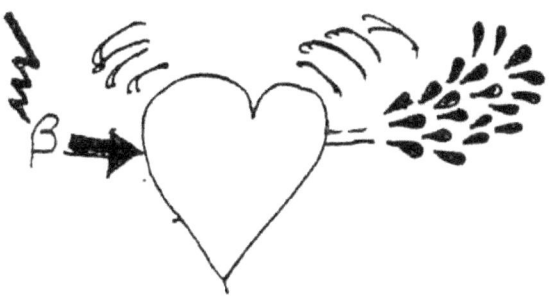

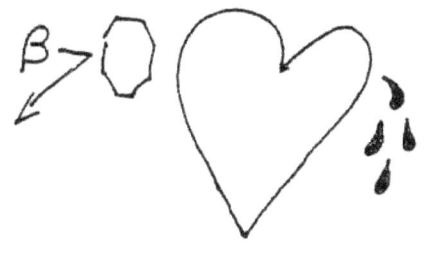

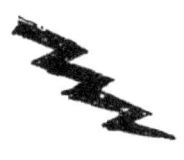

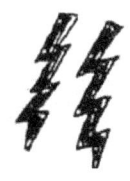

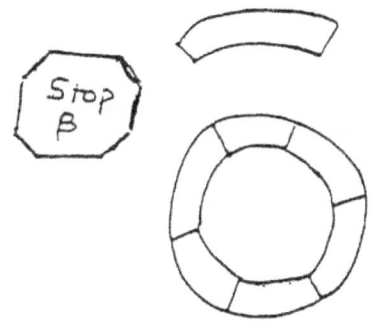

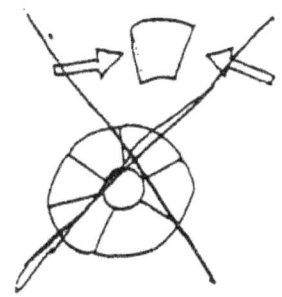

BETA BLOCKERS for HYPERTENSION

For combating hypertension beta blockers are second only to diuretics. Beta blockers reduce the the heart rate and contractility. This produces less blood flow. Beta blockers prevent the sympathetic nervous system from activating the renin-angiotensin system.

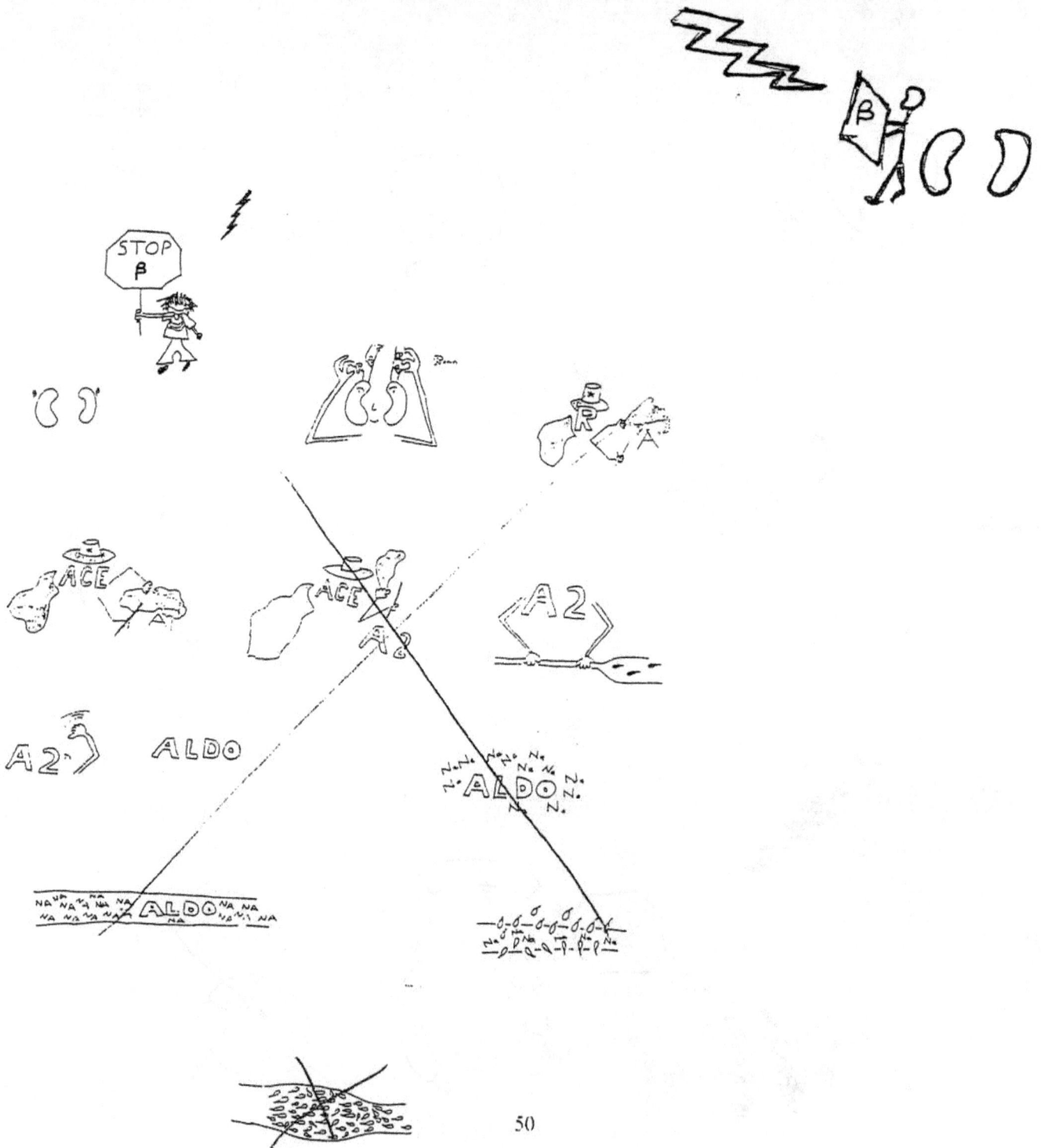

50

CALCIUM CHANNEL BLOCKERS for HYPERTENSION

Calcium channel blockers are very effective blood pressure lowering agents. In addition to their effects on cardiac conduction, they relax vascular smooth muscle which dilate the arteries.

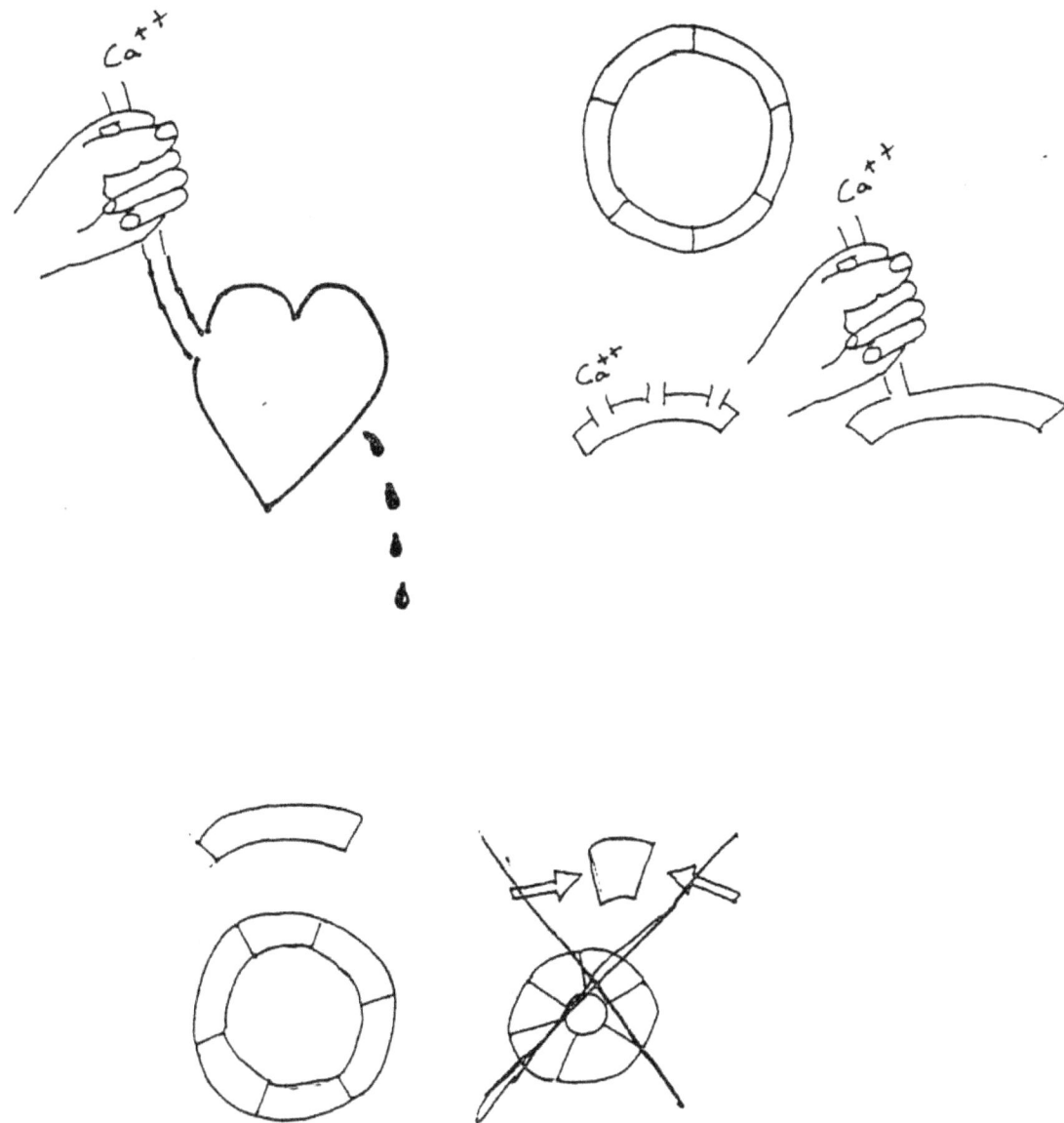

What more can I say?

Types of diuretics:

Thiazide diuretics (Diuril, Zaroxolyn, Hydrodiuril)

Loop diuretics (Lasix, Bumex, Edecrine) In addition to losing water, k,potassium, sodium and calcium is lost. Usually potassium is given with the loop diuretics.

Potassium Sparing Diuretics (Triamterine, Spirolactone) These are given with a thiazide diuretic to counteract the problem of losing potassium.

ANGIOTENSIN RECEPTOR BLOCKERS (ARB)

For hypertension angiotensin receptor blockers have the same result as ace inhibitors. They work in a different place in the renin-angiotensin-aldosterone system. Three examples are Cozaar, Avapro and Diovan. I think the picture shows best what they do.

ANGIOTENSIN RECEPTOR BLOCKERS (ARB)

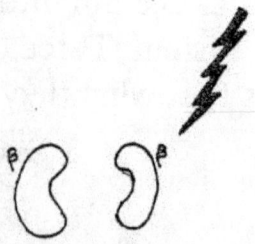

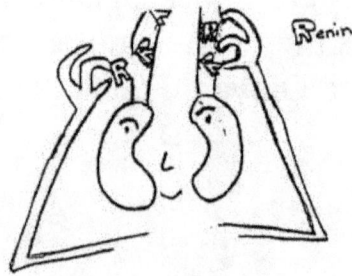

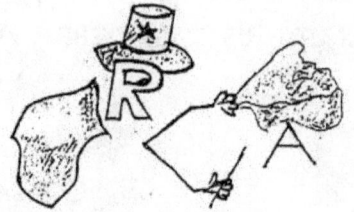

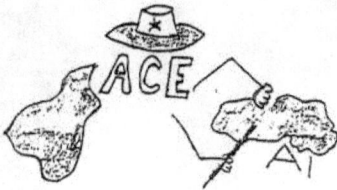

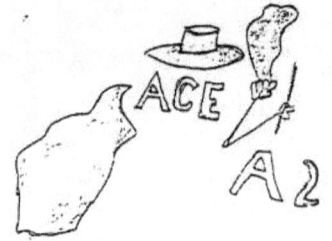

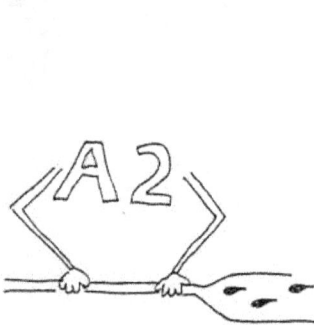

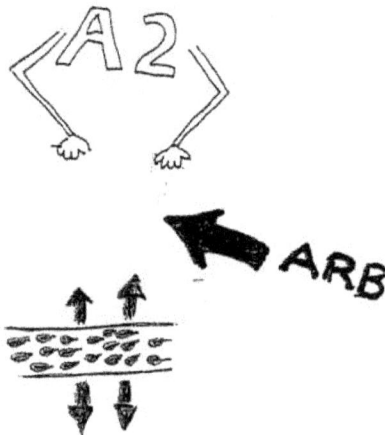

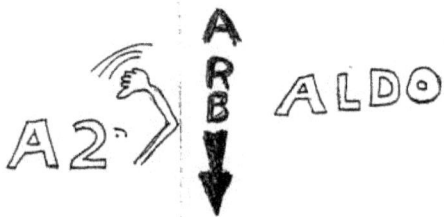

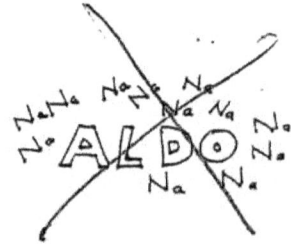

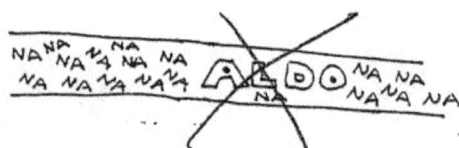

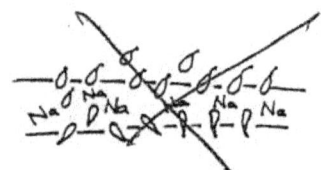

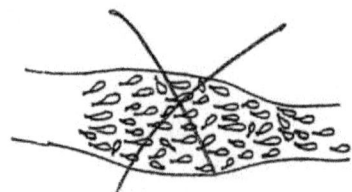

ANGINA

As I may have mentioned, the heart is a muscle. Like any cell muscles get their nutrients and oxygen from red blood cells in the blood.

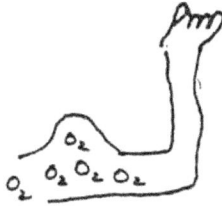

When any muscle contracts vigorously it needs more oxygen.

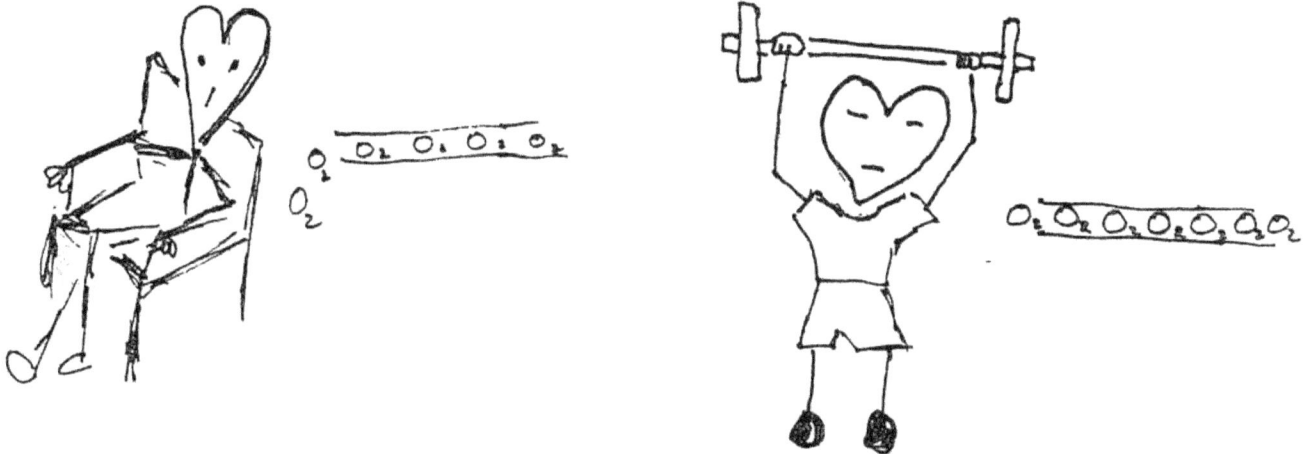

And less oxygen when it contracts less vigorously.

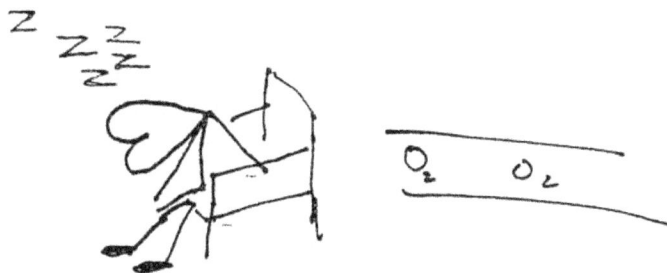

To meet that need blood vessels normally respond by enlarging and supplying more blood for more oxygen. If muscles don't get enough oxygen you feel pain. Leg cramps after exercise is an example of that. A heart not getting enough oxygen feels a pain called angina.

If our guy went from sitting to weight lifting, the extra oxygen would be supplied by the coronary arteries dilating and allowing greater blood flow to the heart muscle.

If an obstruction blocks or limits the flow of blood (and oxygen) that's called coronary artery disease (CAD). This can result in exertional chest pain (angina) or muscle death (myocardial infarction)

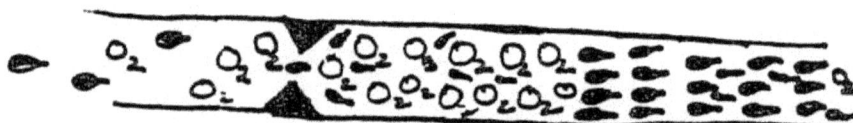

What do we do for that problem? First slow down. That reduces oxygen requirements. If you are working in a hospital that would probably mean getting back to bed (not you, the patient). Giving the patient oxygen would also get more oxygen to the heart.

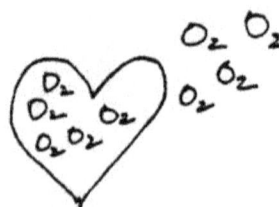

And drugs. Nitroglycerine sublingual is practically synonymous with relief from angina. It might interest you to know that nitroglycerine has been used to treat angina since 1879. Nitroglycerine reduces the oxygen needs of the heart by dilation of the vasculature and dilation of the narrowed coronary artery which allows more blood flow to the heart muscle.

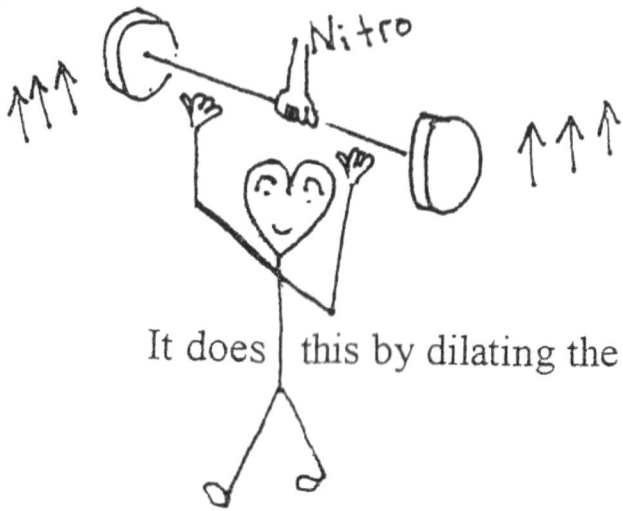

It does this by dilating the body's vasculature.

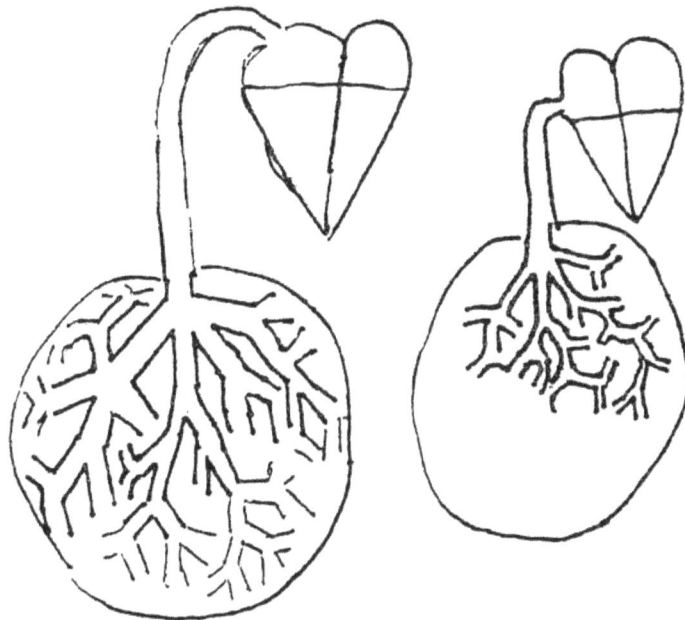

Dilating veins reduces veinous return (preload) to the heart. So there is less blood for the heart to pump. That makes it easier for the heart to pump. It has to contract less vigorously. Thus the heart requires less coronary artery blood flow as a result of the lowered oxygen requirements of the heart.

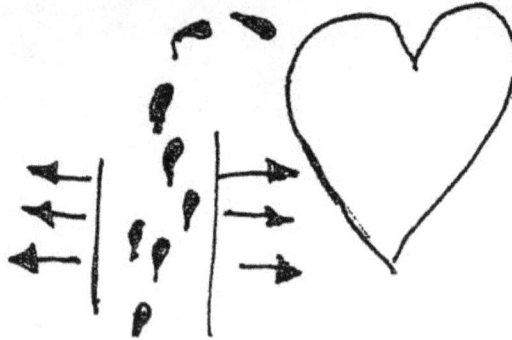

It also works by dilating the coronary arteries and allowing more blood to flow to the heart muscle.

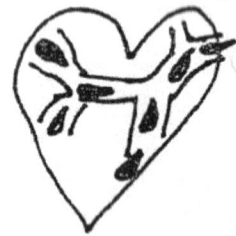

NITRATES for ANGINA and HYPERTENSION

In general nitrates open the veinous side (as opposed to the arterial side) of circulation. There are three reasons for nitrates.

#1 Hypertension. For a hypertensive emergency Nipride I.V. is a potent vasodilator.

#2 Cardiac workload. Following a heart attack it is a good idea to give the heart a break to decrease its need for oxygen. Opening up the vasculature with nitrates is good way.

#3 Cardiac oxygenation. To improve the blood flow to the heart nitrates up the vasculature of the heart. As we said earlier this can be done quickly with with sublingual nitroglycerine. Or it can be done over a longer period with oral nitrates like Isordil or Nitrodur.

BETA BLOCKERS for ANGINA

Beta blockers reduce oxygen demand by slowing the heart at the sinus node and reducing contractility.

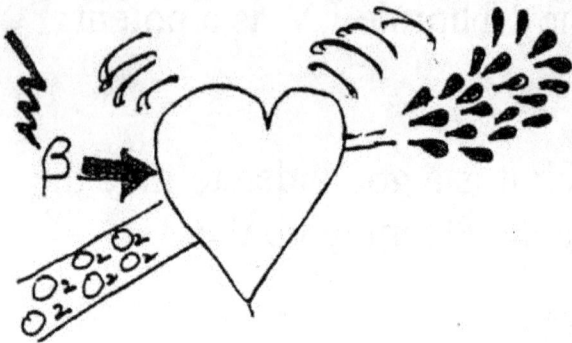

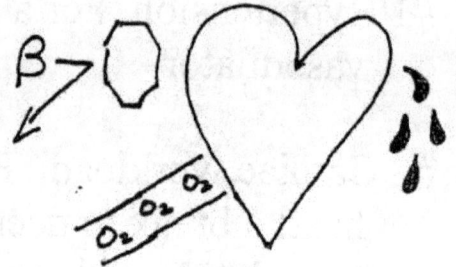

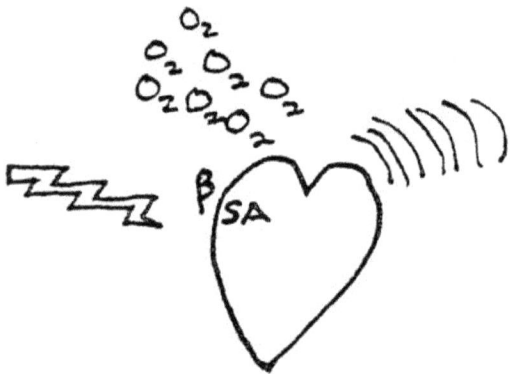

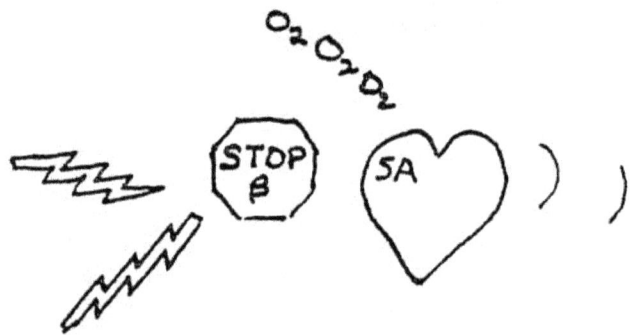

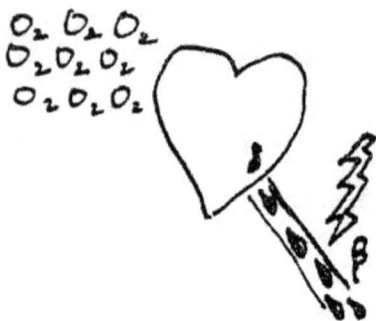

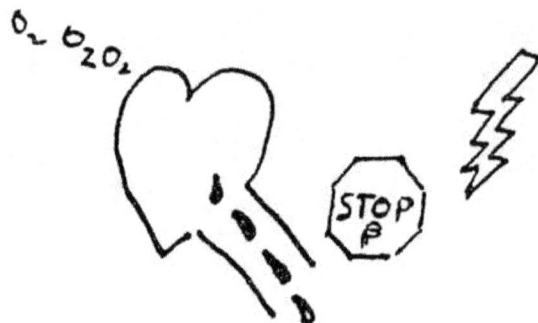

CALCIUM CHANNEL BLOCKERS for ANGINA

Calcium channel blockers work in a way similar to nitrates. They dilate coronary arteries and systemic arteries. They have little effect on veins. Verapamil and diltiazem have the additional benefit of slowing the heart rate (like the beta blockers).

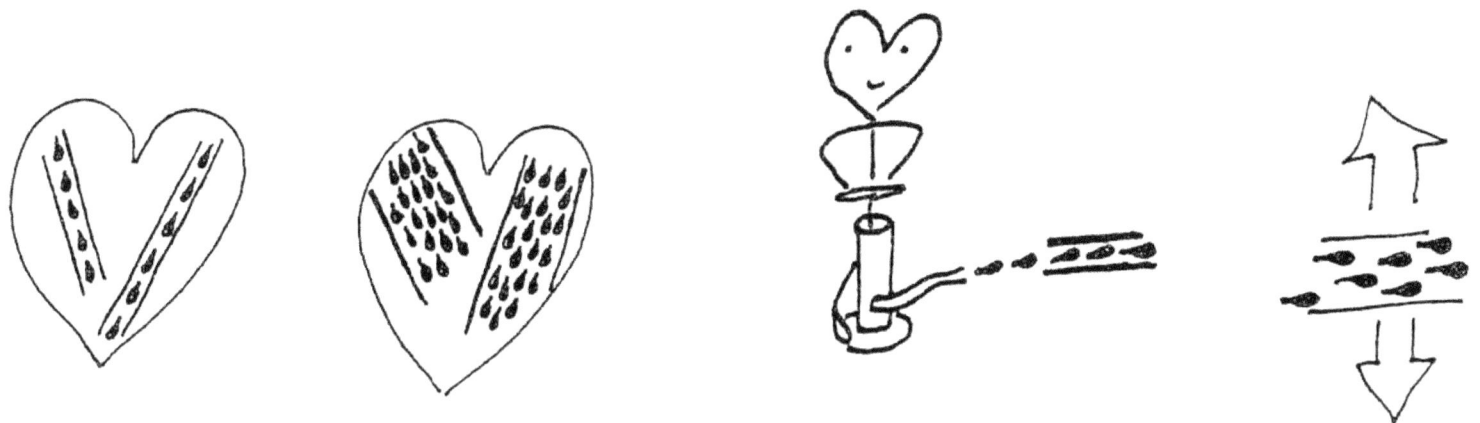

LOW BLOOD PRESSURE

What if you take somebody's blood pressure and its 84/39. You know that's way too low. But why and what do you do about it?

Lets look at the causes. Either the heart is not pumping enough blood (a pump problem), or there isn't enough blood (a volume problem) or the circulatory system has expanded too much (a space problem)

What's the problem with low blood pressure? I mean isn't it good the heart doesn't have to pump so hard for once? It's nice you're giving your heart a break. But your body probably isn't getting enough blood to all the tissues for nourishment. The reason I make that generality is that it is in the tiny capillaries where nutrients cross from the blood to the tissues and where most of the resistance to blood blow occurs. It is blood pressure pushing it through that resistance.

So if you measure low blood pressure, the blood probably isn't being pushed through the tiny capillaries where the tissues get nourished.

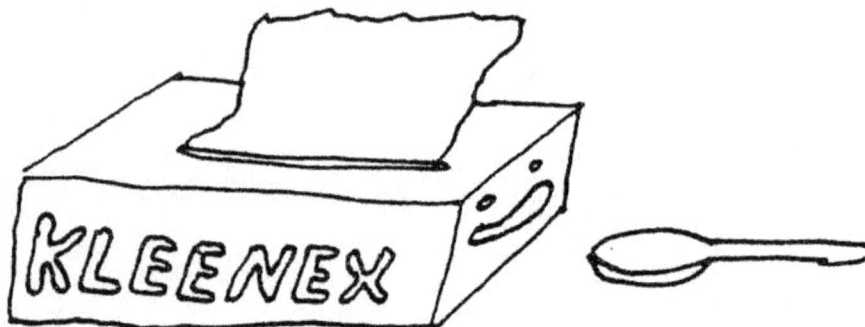

So we've decided that when you get a low blood pressure, the heart isn't pumping enough, or there isn't enough blood or the vasculature has over expanded. What would be the signs and symptoms? Light headed feelings, passing out because the brain isn't getting enough blood. Mottled extremities because they aren't getting perfused. Pale complexion. Impaired mentation, or worse, loss of consciousness because of poor perfusion to the brain.

When you measure excessively low blood pressure the first step would be to lie the patient down. Most likely there isn't enough oomph to lift blood to the highest point in the body (and a very important organ) the brain. It is best to lie them flat or even trendelenberg so the blood gets to the brain and they don't lose consciousness.

We will talk about why the blood pressure is low. But in a critical situation you won't have time to think about that. Listen to the lungs. If they are clear you will give likely push I.V. fluids (unless they are in CHF) and dopamine or other cardiac stimulent.

You would certainly call the doctor. Depending on your hospital's and your particular floor's protocol you might call for a stat EKG and a stat chest x-ray.

Once the patient is stabilized you may want to determine the cause. This will be especially important when the doctor calls back. The I/O is a place to start.

If the patient has a fever and elevated WBC count could guess septic shock. Septic shock is a vascular response to e choli, shigella other gram negative bugs. All blood vessels dilate. There is a huge increase in the vascular space. Fluids would be the most pointed response. For the choice of cardiac stimulant you would want more alpha (periferal vasoconstriction) than beta 1 (increased cardiac output). A good vasopressor is norepinepherine (levophed). For pure alpha stimulation, there is phenylepherine or Neo-Synephrine. It only causes vasoconstriction. You may know it as an over the counter medication for for nasal congestion. It shrinks swollen nasal mucus membranes.

If the patient has low fluid intake, poor skin turgor and labs indicating dehydration you could guess hypovolemia. Look for a high BUN/creatinine ratio. Fluids would address this problem.

CONDUCTION SYSTEM

The best way to begin the section on the conduction system is to imagine this scenario: 3:00 A.M. The monitor shows a heart rate of 150 beats a minute. The patient is asymtomatic. You call the doctor. You probably know the response. Either digoxin 0.125-0.250 mg or verapamil 2.5-5 mg. And a twelve lead EKG. We'll go on to see that as a pure conduction situation.

The cardiac conduction system is a bundle of wires that delivers a little shock to each of the muscle fibers of the heart in an orderly sequence. How was that for a definition?

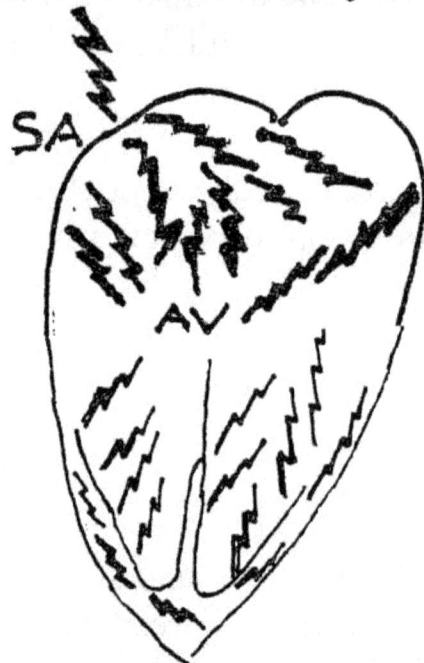

It is needed so the timing impulse for heart contraction is rapidly spread to both atria so that they can contract in unison.

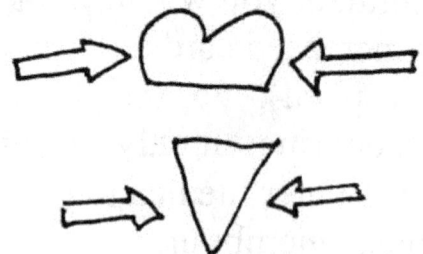

The conduction system delays the impulse so the ventricles have time to fill before they contract. Then they both contract in unison.

The conduction system is the SA node, the AV node, the bundle of His, the left and right branches and the fibers of Purkinje.

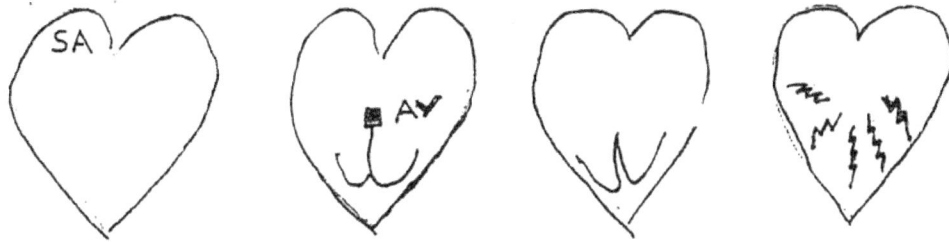

The S.A. node is in the right upper corner of the right atrium. At this point in the cardiac sequence, blood has filled both atria. Next about 75% of the blood passively falls through the tricuspid and mitral valves into the right and left ventricles. The S.A. node fires a small electrical charge. The charge propagates through both atria. It stimulates each muscle cell to contract. After each cell contracts, the charge is transmitted to the next muscle cell. It takes about 0.06 seconds to complete the propagation through both atria.

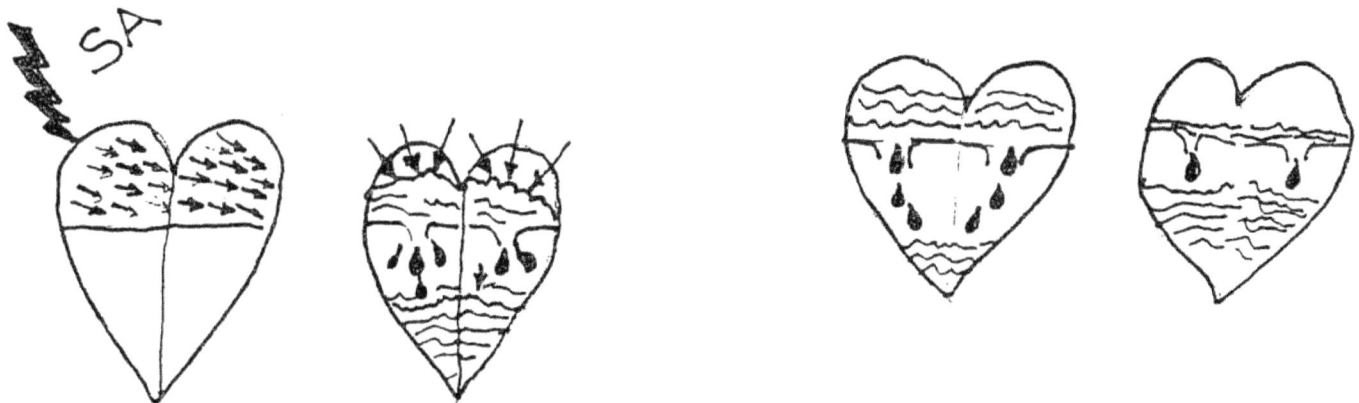

The impulse travels through both atria to the A.V. (atrioventricular) node.

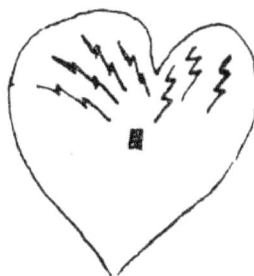

On the way to the ventricles the A.V. node delays the impulse $1/10$ of a second.

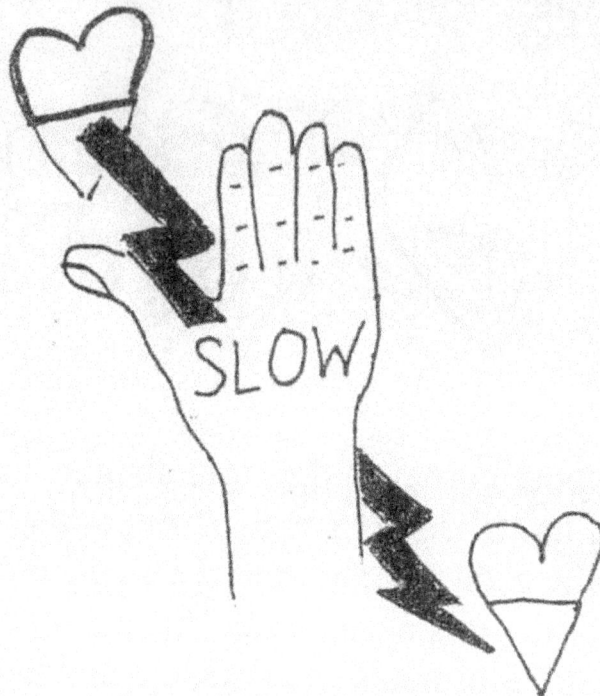

That gives the ventricles time to fill before they begin to contract.

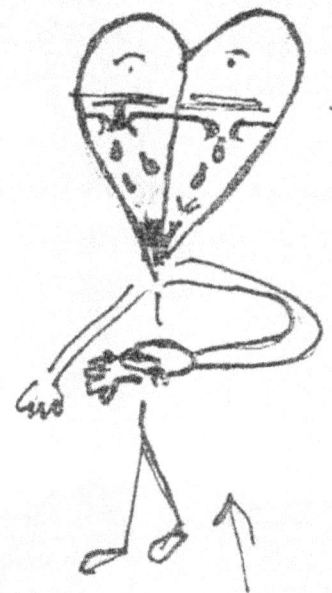

The A.V. node is make of conductive tissue just like the S.A. node. The A.V. node slows down the impulse because of its smaller diameter.

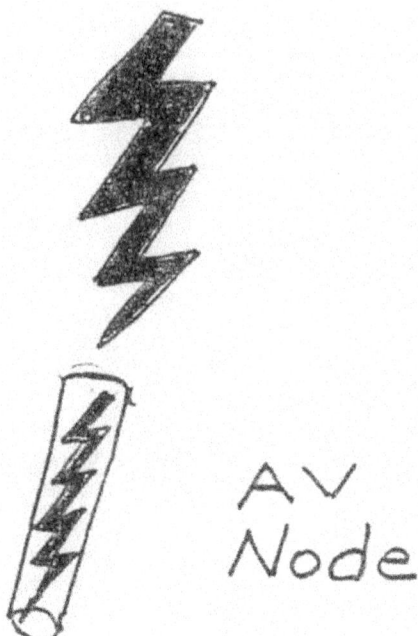

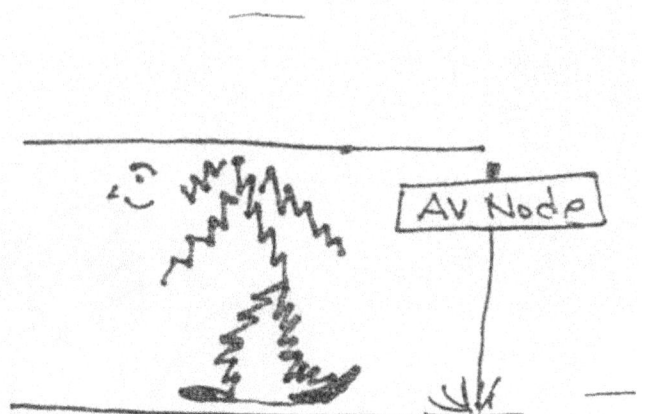

AV
Node

After the impulse has passed through the
A.V. node it continues along the conduction
pathway. Next it enters the bundle of His.

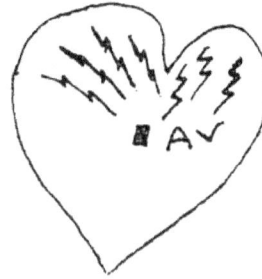

The ventricular conduction system divides into
The left and right bundle branches.

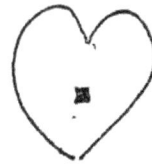

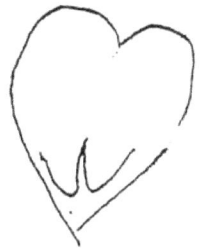

These branches further subdivide into
Numerous Purkinje fibers.

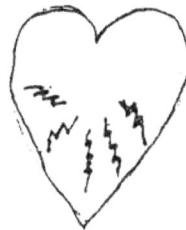

Finally the Purkinje fibers make contact with myocardial cells in the
ventricles. Then the contraction and electrical charge spread from muscle
fiber to adjacent muscle fiber. You see this electrical charge as the QRS
wave on an EKG.

SYMPATHETIC & PARASYMPATHETIC
CONTROL of HEART RATE

The S.A. node and the A.V. nodes are controlled by the sympathetic and parasympathetic nervous system. The sympathetic system aimed at the S.A. node increases the rate of firing. The parasympathetic (sometimes called vagal) system slows down the rate of firing. In the picture the rabbit is the sympathetic and the turtle is the parasympathetic. The sympathetic receptors are beta 1. So a sympathetic stimulation of the S.A. node would make it fire its impulses at a faster rate.

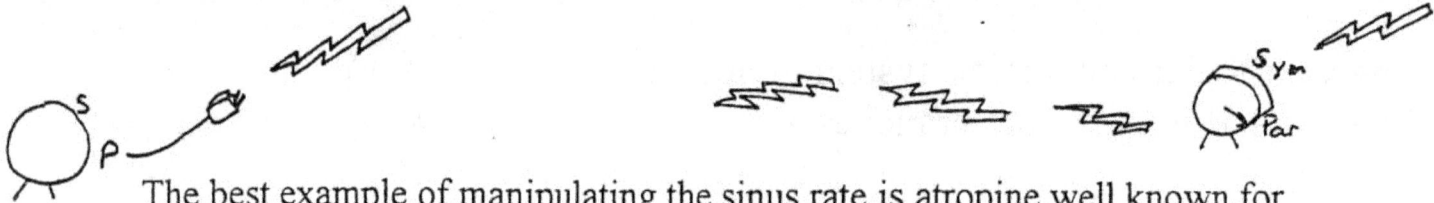

The best example of manipulating the sinus rate is atropine well known for bradycardia. Atropine squelches the parasympathetic system. That gives the sympathetic system free reign to speed up the firing rate.

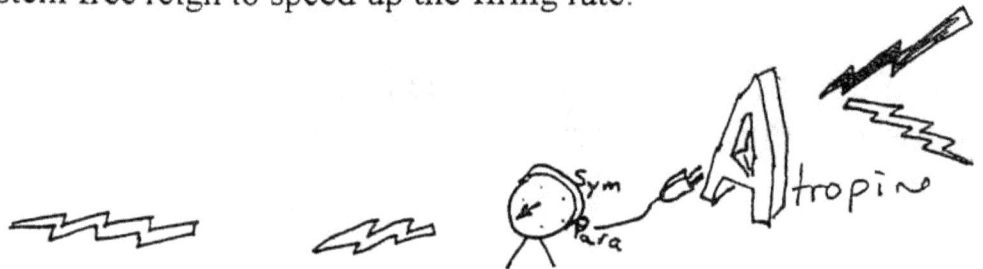

The sympathetic and parasympathetic systems also regulate transmission through the A.V. node. Parasympathetic stimulation makes transmission through the A.V. node slower

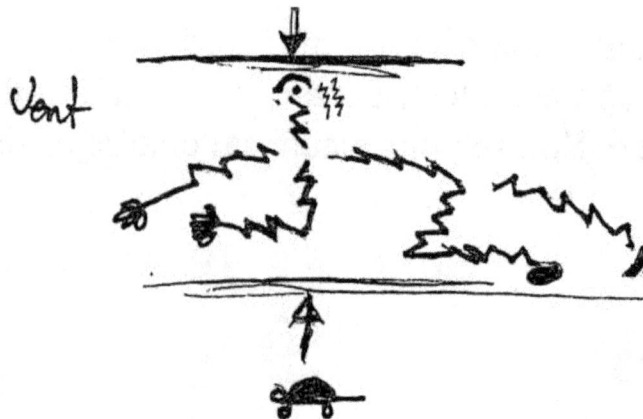

And sympathetic stimulation makes transmission through the A.V. node faster.

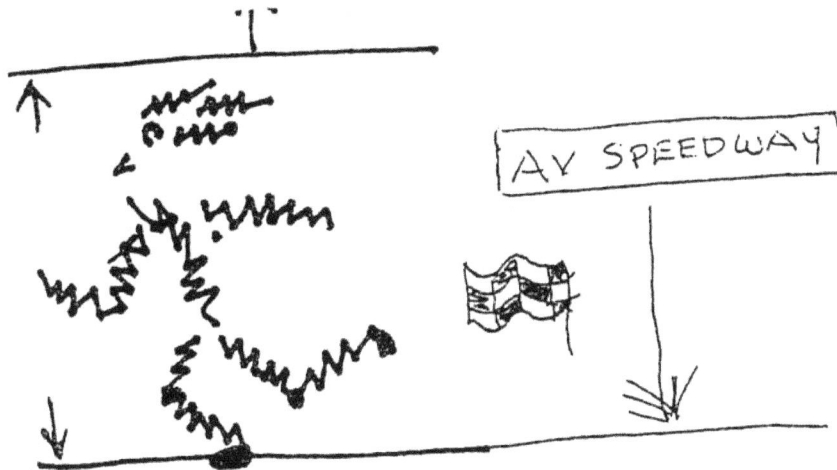

CONDUCTIVE TISSUE

The "wires" or "conduction pathways" we have been talking about are conduction tissues. Conduction tissue is only slightly different from regular heart muscle cells. In the next picture we see a familiar sight: the response of a heart muscle cell to a stimulus. The electrolytes move in and out. The cell contracts and transmits the electrical impulse to the adjacent cell.

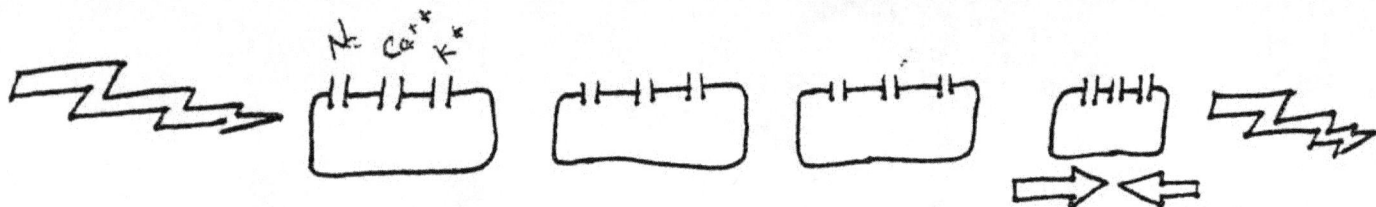

The conduction cell is the same except that it does not contract.

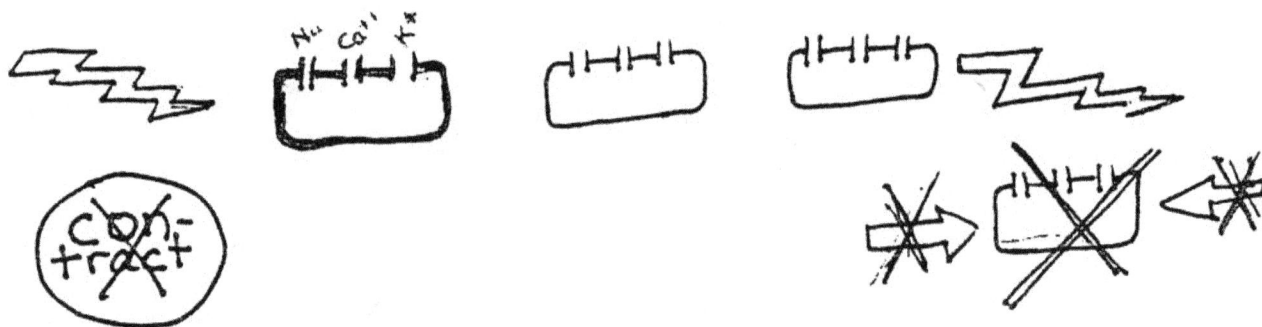

We will soon learn that most drugs for conduction problems are aimed at controlling the electrolyte transfers.

AUTOMATICITY

Automaticity is another important feature of the conduction system. Automaticity is the ability to spontaneously fire an electrical charge. Every cell in the conduction system can do that. The SA node, the AV node, the bundle branches and Purkinje fibers can all spontaneously fire an electrical charge. Mostly they are at a regular rate - like your normal heart rate. Sometimes they are not regular - like when your heart "skips a beat" or "goes pitter patter".

SA Node

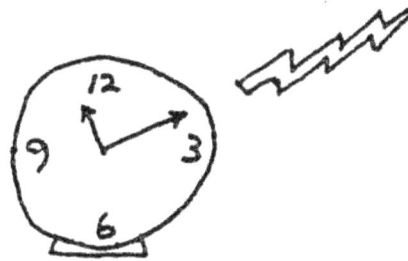

Normally the electrical charge begins in the SA node. **Automaticity** is the SA node's ability to spontaneously depolorize. Said in other words, the SA node starts the electrical charge. Or in a picture:

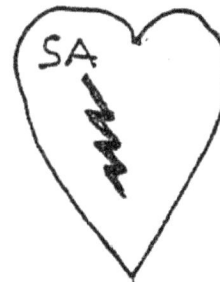

Of all the conduction tissue, the SA node has the capacity for firing the fastest. That's why fires normally, it overrides the other sites. That is to say the Sa node paces the entire heart. Should the SA node fail to fire, other sites in the conduction system will take over pacing of the heart – but usually at a slower rate.

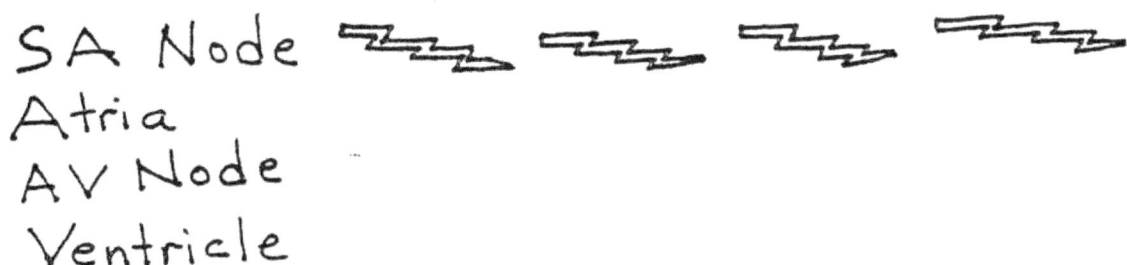

SA Node
Atria
AV Node
Ventricle

TOO MUCH AUTOMATICITY

Sometimes a misbehaving cell can fire on its own. That's called ectopic focus. If it happens in the atria, it's called a **premature atrial contraction.**

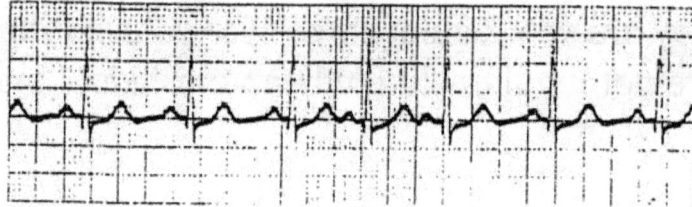

If it happens in the ventricles, it's called a **premature ventricular contraction.**

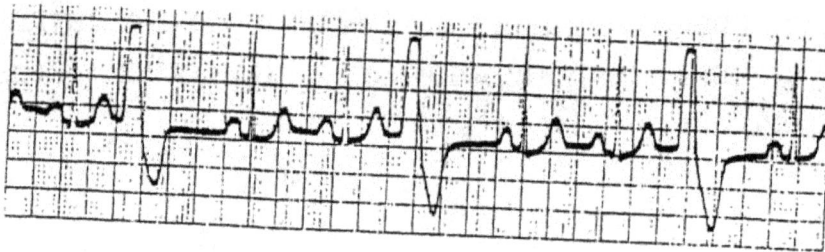

In both cases the atria and ventricles contract. But since they havent't had time to fill with blood they are ejecting less than a full atria or ventricle. Thus less blood is ejected with each premature beat.

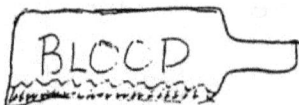

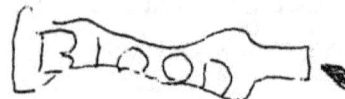

Things can get worse. There are three arrhythmias of the atria that are lumped together as **supraventricular.** Supraventricular means above the ventricles. They are supraventricular tachycardia, atrial flutter and atrial fibrillation. They are all some form of automaticity that occurs in the atria.

Supraventricular tachycardia **one** ectopic focus in the atria firing at a rate if 150 to 250 beats a minute. The rate is fast but constant – in other words the same spacing between each beat on an EKG.

Atrial flutter is atrial flutter is similar – except faster, 250 to 350 beats per minute. You can easily recognize the saw-tooth EKG. Notice the spacing is constant

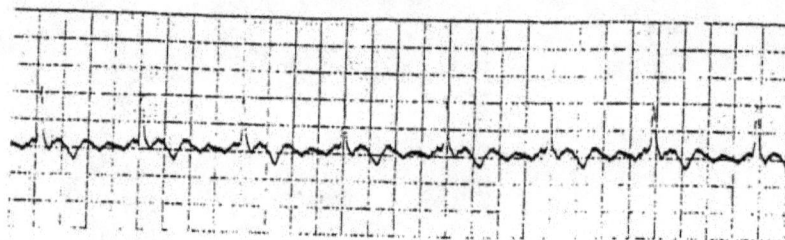

Atrial fibrillation is caused by multiple ecctopic foci firing at random. This shows up on the EKG as unevenly spaced different heights.

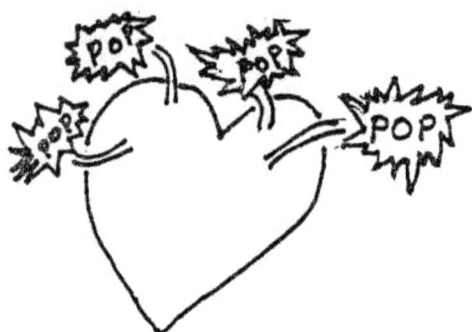

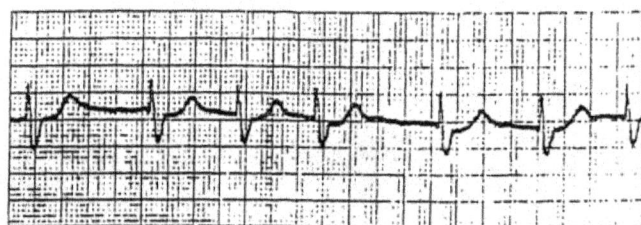

If flushing the toilet before the tank fills doesn't move much water, what happens when you compulsively jiggle the handle? What does happen is that the atrial contraction is lost. But that only accounts for the last 25% of the blood being squeezed out after the first 75% has fallen through the valves. So the heart is still probably moving enough blood. The major risk is that slower moving blood can coagulate and form clots. To treat this Coumadin is prescribed.

DRUGS FOR SUPRAVENTRICULAR TACHYCARDIA

DIGOXIN for SUPRAVENTRICULAR TACHYCARDIA

For atrial fibrillation and flutter, **digoxin** is frequently prescribed. Digoxin does not abolish the arrhythmia. It strengthens the parasympathetic (vagal) tone and thereby slows conduction through the AV node. That decreases the number of impulses reaching the ventricles. That way the ventricles can pump at a slower, more efficient rate. Increasing the parasympathetic tone also does what to the SA node? Remember the turtle?

It slows the rate the SA node fires. That is why you must count the pulse and never give digoxin if the rate is less than 60 beats per minute.

You must also check the potassium level. A low potassium level potentiates the effect of digoxin. Digoxin has a small therapeutic range. That means a small increase in serum levels can cause a toxic effect. Dig interferes with the exchange of calcium and potassium. This will be important in the next section on CHF.

CALCIUM CHANNEL BLOCKERS for
SUPRAVENTRICULAR TACHYCARDIA

Calcium channel blockers are called class IV antiarrhythmics. Verapamil (Calan, Isoptin) is the drug of choice for supraventricular tachycardia. Cardizem follows. They slow the rate of calcium intake. That slows the rate the impulse can be transmitted through the AV node.

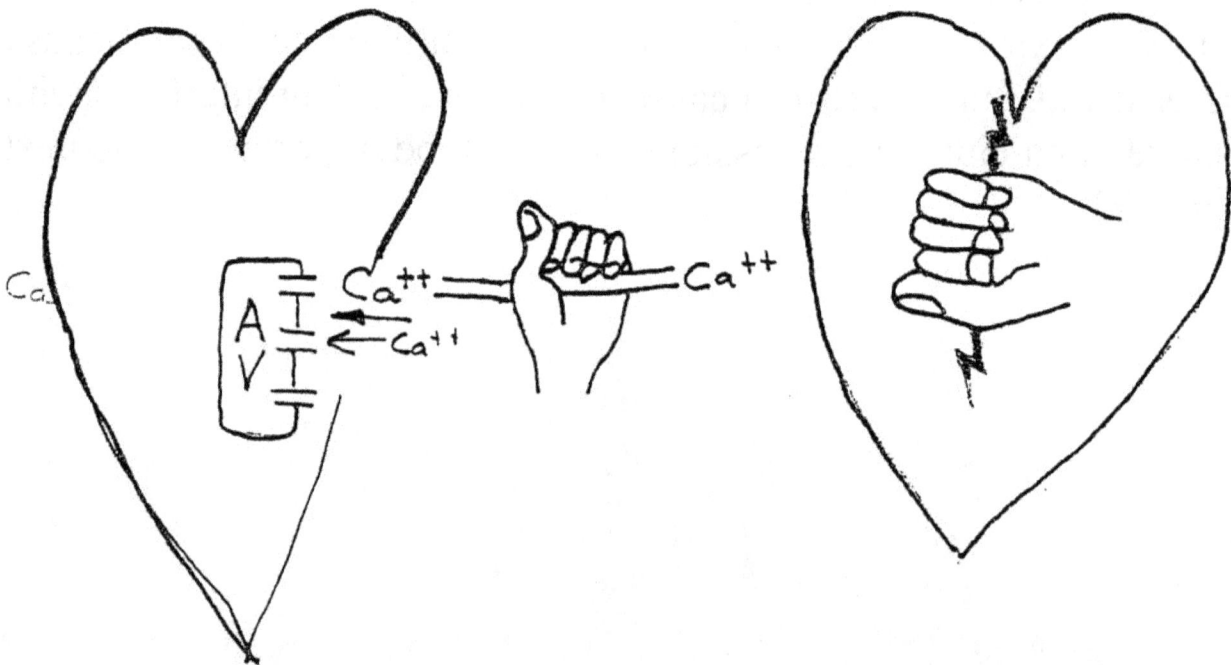

BETA BLOCKERS FOR SUPRAVENTRICULAR TACHYCARDIA

Beta blockers are called class II antiarrhythmics. Beta blockers block the sympathetic response to the AV node which slows conduction of the impulse through the AV node.

VENTRICULAR ARRHYTHMIAS
(They are worse than atrial arrhythmias)

They are worse because the ventricles pump the blood.

We already saw one ventricular arrhythmia – premature ventricular contractions. It is one ectopic focus, one deviant conduction cell firing on its own. It decreases the pumping volume of blood because the ventricle hasn't had time to fill. The normally conducted sinus beat leaves time to fill but the premature ventricular contraction does not.

If that same deviant cell really takes off on its own, its called ventricular tachycardia. It looks like this on an EKG.

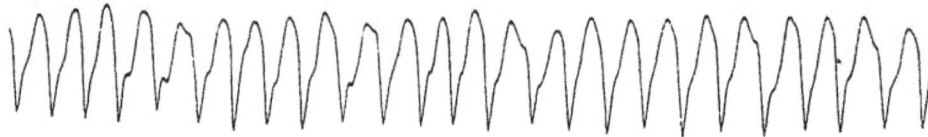

The ventricles are not filling and the pumping is very inefficient. The patient may or may not be stable. The biggest problem is that the sinus node has lost control. There is a big possibility that it may degenerate into ventricular fibrillation.

DRUGS

LIDOCAINE FOR VENTRICULAR TACHYCARDIA

What do we do? We want to squelch that naughty firecracker. We can slow it down so the sinus can take over…with an antiarrhythmic. Most likely lidocaine. Lidocaine is a sodium channel blocker (class I antiarrythmic). Lets look at that misbehaving cell under a microscope.

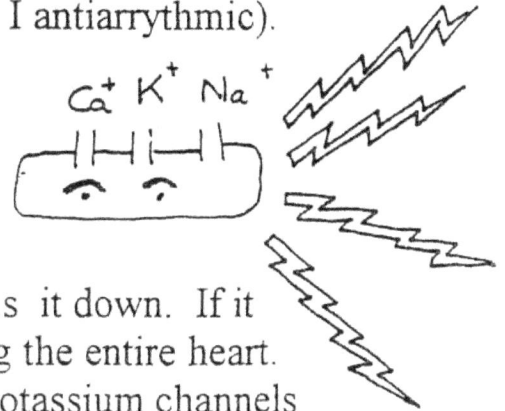

Lidocaine blocks the sodium channel and just s..l..o..w..s it down. If it slows down enough, the sinus node can take over pacing the entire heart. If lidocaine doesn't work, bretylium is next. It blocks potassium channels the same way lidocaine blocks the sodium channels or verapamil blocks the calcium channels.

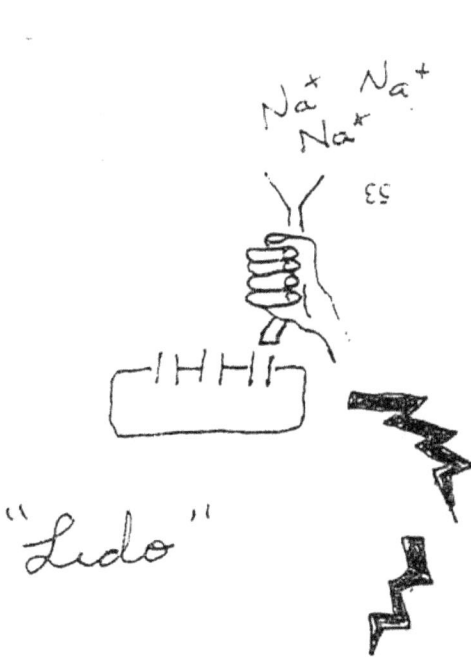

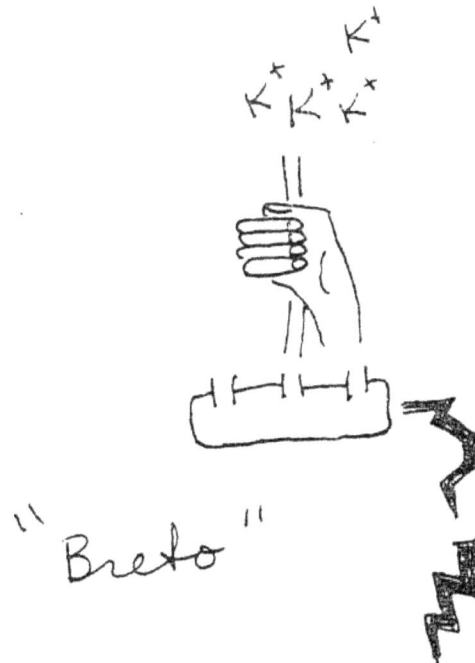

"Lido"

"Breto"

V-FIB...CODE BLUE

Ventricular fibrillation is numerous ectopic foci all firing in total disarray.

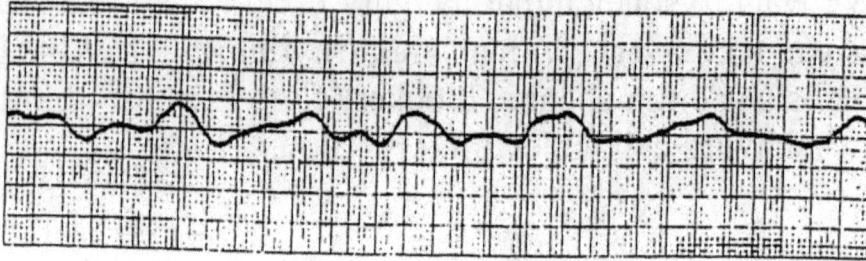

The net result is that the ventricles just quiver. No blood moves. The patient has minutes to live.

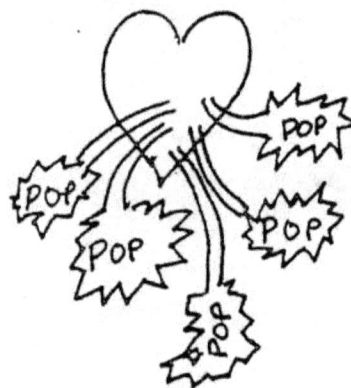

CONGESTIVE HEART FAILURE

Congestive heart failure is heart failure. The heart can't pump enough blood to meet the body's needs. The most obvious symptom is fatigue. Shortness of breath is caused by fluid in the lungs. Leg swelling is caused by veinous engorgement in the legs and weight gain from fluid retention. It is called congestive because blood tends to back up in distended jugular veins and other veins causing ankle edema (another frequent sign). The most frequent cause is the damage from a heart attack. The local area of dead heart tissue can't contract and the overall pumping is impaired. Other causes of CHF are hypertension, viral infections, arrhythmias and aging.

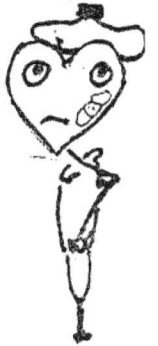

Once the heart has started to pump less blood another series of events begins that must be reversed. The body senses (in the baroreceptors in the aorta) lower blood flow. It thinks the body just suffered a major blood loss.

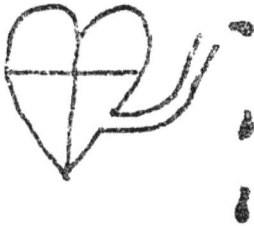

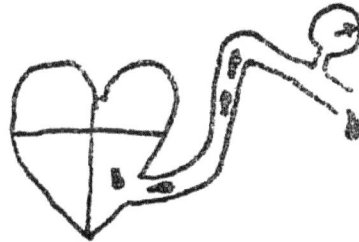

It activates the central nervous system and adrenal glands.

Given a perception of less blood volume the sympathetic nervous system and adrenals try to redirect blood flow to major organs. It does this by increasing peripheral resistance by way of epinephrine and norepinepherine.

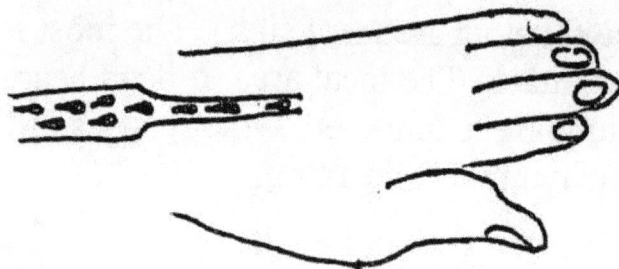

Unfortunately the heart must pump against greater vascular resistance. To an already failing heart this could likely cause further decline.

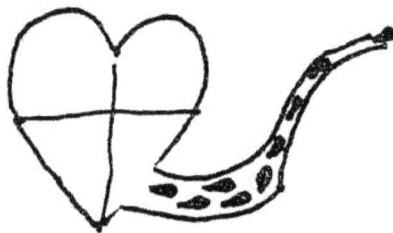

As you doubtless remember (from page   ) what else the sympathetic nervous system does when it perceives less blood volume.

It activates the kidneys. It activates the renin angiotensin which clamps down on the vasculature. And aldosterone causes retention of sodium which causes retention of water.

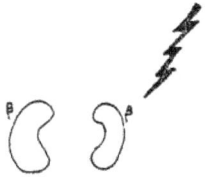

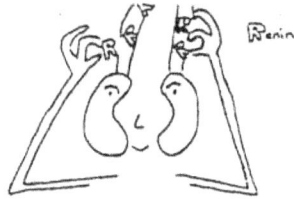

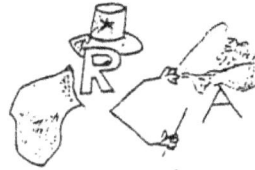

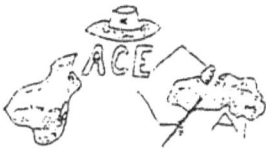

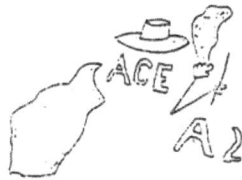

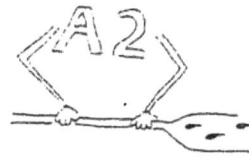

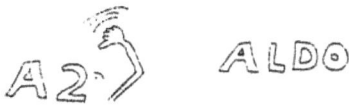

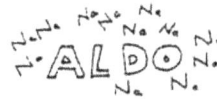

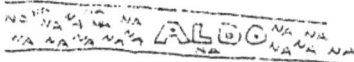

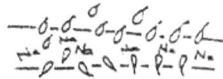

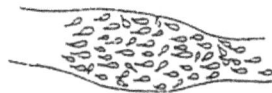

So the heart has to pump more volume against more resistance.

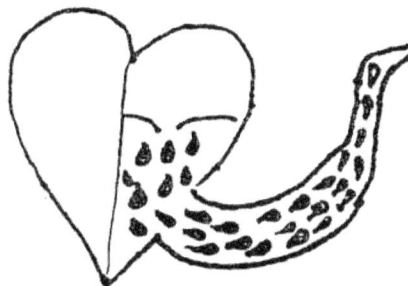

Things get worse. The kidneys receive reduced blood flow because the heart is pumping less. That in itself causes less fluid to be eliminated as urine.

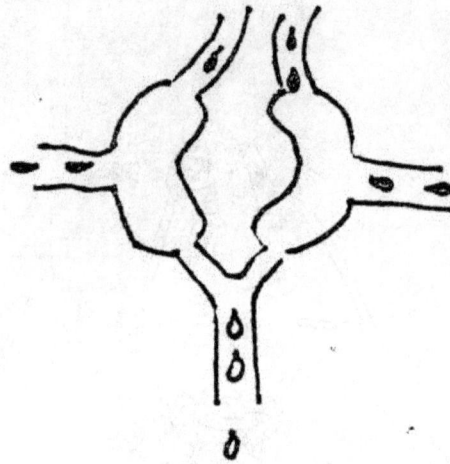

So...The injured heart is pumping more fluid against greater resistance.

That's what causes the edema. If the right side of the heart fails, edema will likely show up in the ankles and jugular veins.

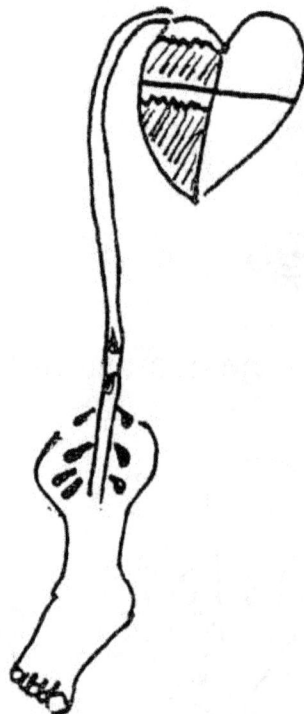

Three things are causing this.

There is more fluid.

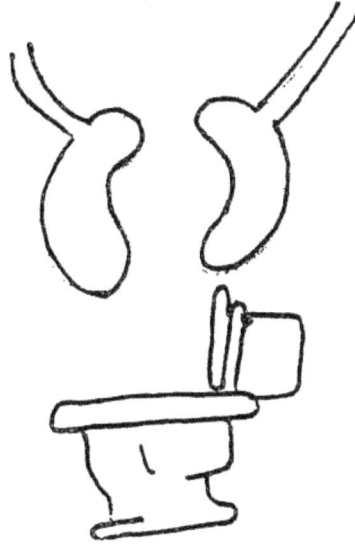

The capillaries are under greater pressure and fluid flows out of them into the tissues.

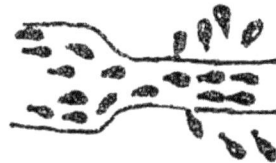

And the blood is backing up because the heart is not able to pump all that gets to it.

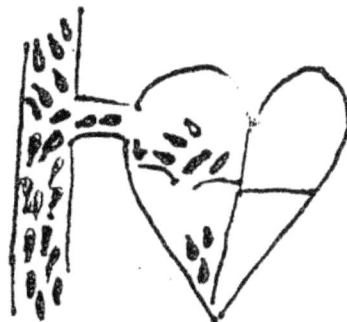

If the left side of the heart fails the edema is in the lungs. That is called pulmonary edema. The most obvious sign is pink frothy sputum. The combination of vasoconstriction, more volume, and blood backing up causes fluid to leak out into the alveoli via the pulmonary cappilaries.

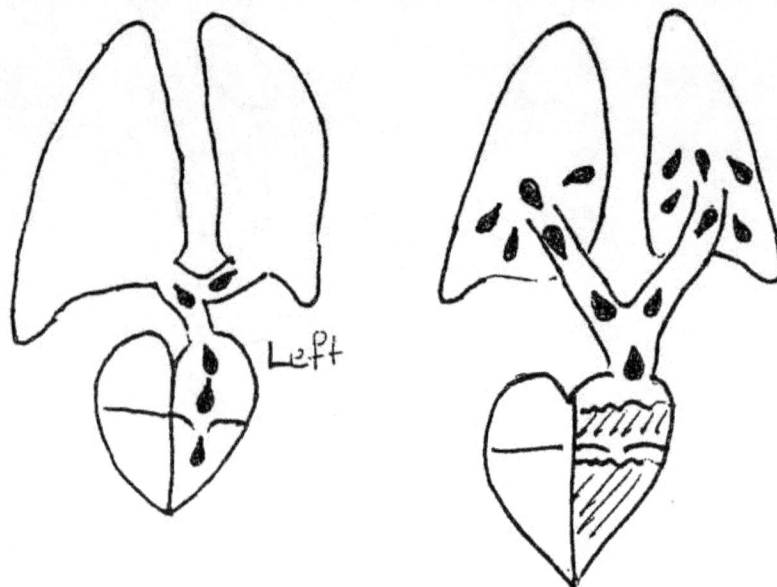

The alveoli of course are the microscopic sacs where oxygen diffuses into the blood from the lungs and carbon dioxide does the opposite. Fluid backing up into the alveoli will make its way into the sputum. We call that condition pulmonary edema – edema in the lungs. That is probably the best known sign of left sided heart failure.

If uncorrected pulmonary edema leads to further oxygen deficit.

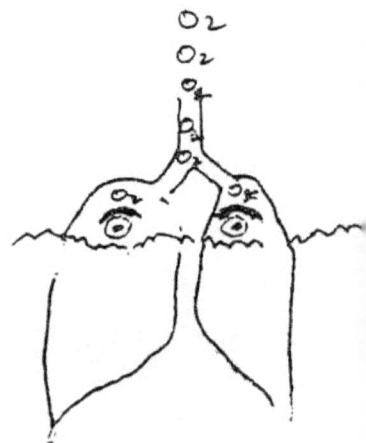

What can we do? The first step is to reverse the weak contractions with inotropic agents. Dopamine and dobutamine are beta 1 stimulators that enhance myocardial contractility. But they can only be given by I.V. infusion. Amrinone is a new inotropic agent. (phospho   inhibitor) which also increases the force of contraction of the heart.

DIGOXIN FOR CONGESTIVE HEART FAILURE

While the patient is in the hospital, I.V. inotropic agents like dopamine and dobutamine can be used. But unless the I.V. tubing is very long the benefits are limited to the hospital. So....

Digoxin. For chronic congestive heart failure, the most frequently prescribed drug is digoxin. It strengthens contractions. Digoxin (lanoxin) increases the amount of calcium in the cell.

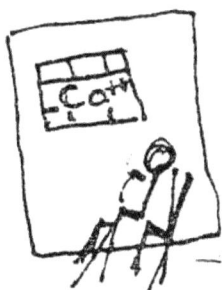

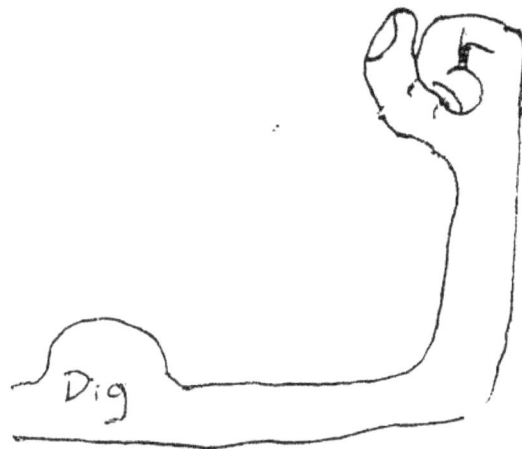

The two most important considerations when giving "dig" ("lan") are heart rate and potassium level. The slower heart rate is slower conduction through the A.V. node. Increased vagal stimulation slows the sinus rate. The importance of potassium is due to $Na+/K+$ - ATPase. You remember that it pushes out sodium and brings in potassium to restore calcium levels. That is why you must know the potassium level before giving dig".

DIURETICS FOR CONGESTIVE HEART FAILURE

Diuretics. We saw the two ways C.H.F. causes fluid retention. (1) Reduced blood flow through the kidneys causes less urine production and (2) How aldosterone promotes retention of sodium which causes water to be retained. The answer in a word: diuretics.

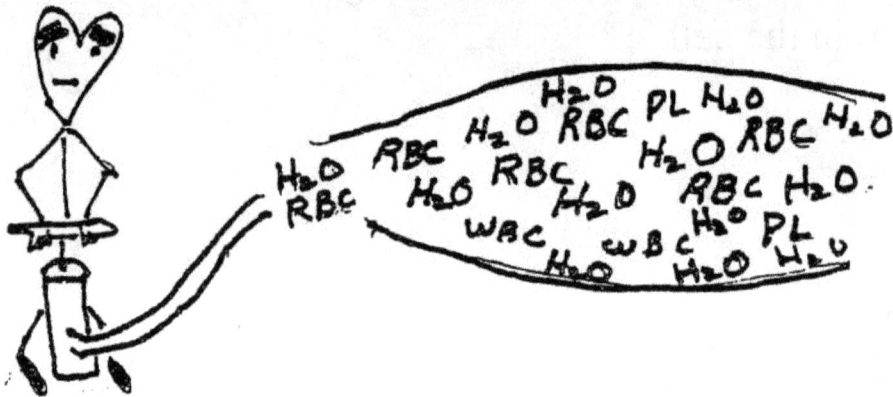

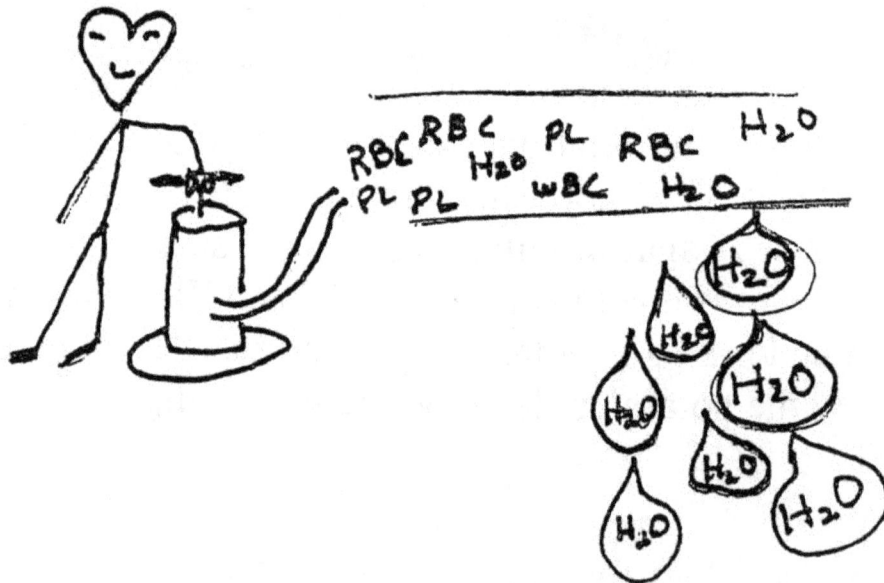

Vasodilators. The other major intervention is vasodilators. Drugs that dilate **arteries** reduce the pressure that the heart must pump against. That is called reducing the afterload.

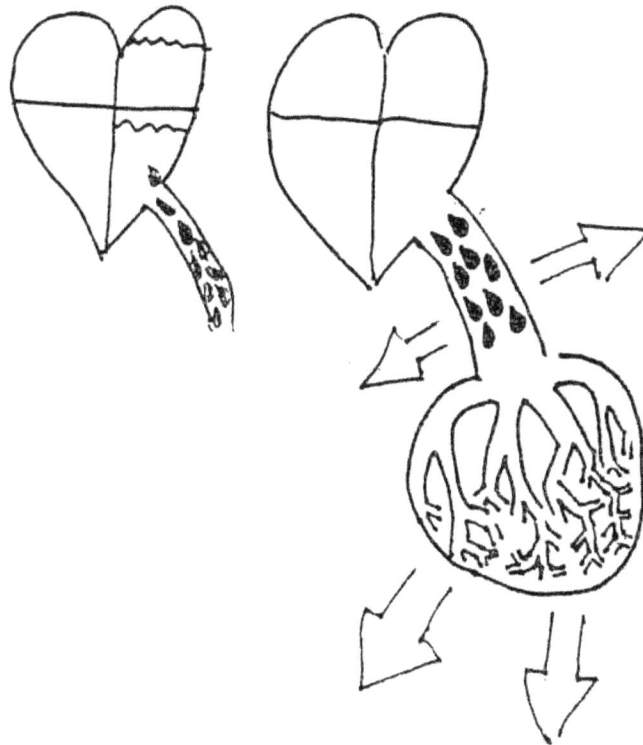

Drugs that dilate **veins** cause less blood to be returned to the heart. That of course means the heart has to pump less blood. That is called reducing the preload. Nitrates and Ace inhibitors dilate the veins.

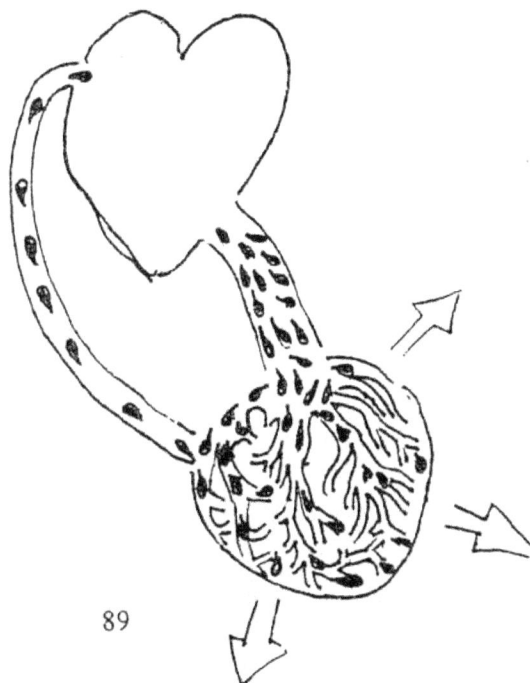

89

DEFIBRILLATION

You all know, "Shock Shock Shock Epi Shock Shock Shock Epi...." This scenario is usually a response to ventricular fibrillation. Ventricular fibrillation is rapid and uncoordinated ventricular impulses that leave the ventricles almost motionless.

Every Ectopic Node fires at SAME TIME

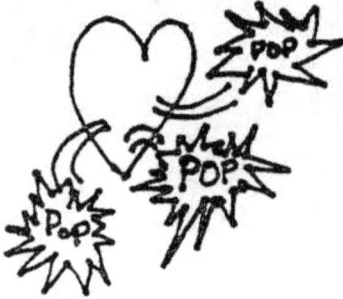

can be settled by

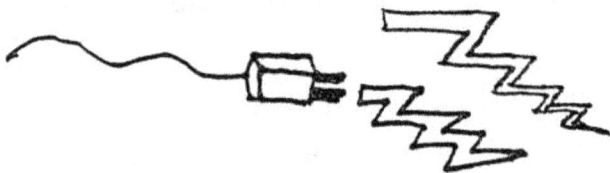

ZAP

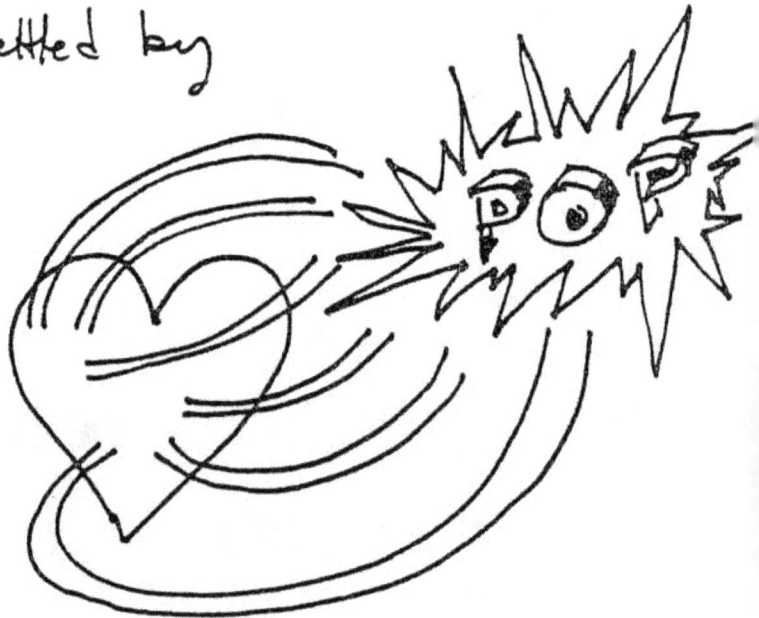

Shocking wipes the slate clean.

And then epinephrine with its beta 1 stimulation inhances the sinus impulse to recapture dominance of the conduction system.

So the sinus node can start

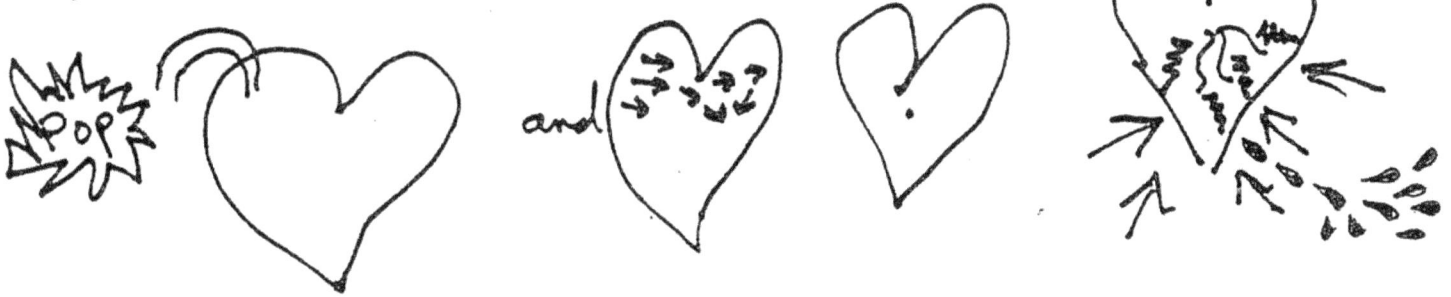

and

CARDIOVERSION

If the arrythmias are atria, either atrial fibrillation or supraventricular tachycardia,

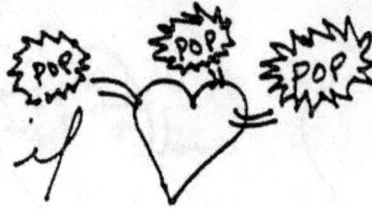

the ZAP ⚡ WILL WAIT FOR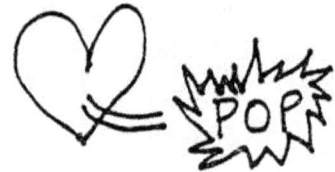

to finish

In other words the electrical impulse will wait for the ventricle to depolarize. In the case of ventriclular fibrillation it doesn't matter when the charge happens. But if the ventricle is beating normally, shocking at the wrong time can put the heart into v-fib (R on T phenomenon). In other words you must use a synchronized shock when converting Afib or SVT.

MEDICAL JOKES

Cardiac Joke: What do you get when you spill a urinal?
Answer: see bottom of page

Immunology Joke: "I'm allergic to lasix. It makes me pee."

Hematology Joke: A vampire goes into a blood bank and asks for one unit of packed red cells and one unit of fresh frozen plasma. The phlebotomist yells back to the tech, "Gimme a Blud and a Blud Lite."

Otolaryngology Joke. For otitis media the doctor ordered "corticosporin drops in the R ear QID" The pharmacist called back to say corticosporin doesn't come in suppository form.

Orthopedic Joke (told by an infectious disease doctor): What do you need to do to pass the orthopedic boards? Be able to bench 200 pounds and spell Ancef.

Urology Joke: The doctor is doing a prostate exam. The guy yells, "That hurts!"
The doctor says," I'm using two fingers."
"Why?"
"I want a second opinion."

Infectious Disease Joke: How do you get a Kleenex to dance? Put a little boogie in it.

C.V. Joke: Did you hear about the two red blood cells who loved in vein?

To impress someone try saying, a gram of acetaminocin instead of two extra strength Tylenols.

G.I. Cartoon: There is a doctor, a nurse and a patient. The patient is draped and in the jack knife position presumabley for a sigmoidoscopy.. The nurse is holding a tray with a bottle of beer. The doctor with an angry look says, "No, I said I wanted a butt light."

I.C.U. Cartoon: There is a patient in an I.C.U. bed with monitors , dynamaps, oxygen, and all the familiar paraphanalia. He is talking on the phone saying, "Bells are ringing and the T.V. has a straight line."

A guy goes in to see a doctor. He touches his head and says, every time I touch it here it hurts." He touches his stomach and says the same thing. He touches his knee and repeats it again. The doctor examines him and says, "Your finger is broken."

Answer to cardiology joke: You get a Pee Wave

A very attractive young man and a vivacious young lady meet in a fashionable night club and they hit it off immediately. Later in the evening they discuss spending the night together and leave immediately for the woman's apartment. As they are getting ready for bed the woman goes into the bathroom and starts to compulsively wash her hands for an excessive length of time. The man asks, "Are you a doctor?"

"Yes."

"Don't tell me! A surgeon! Right?"

"Yes. How did you know?"

"It was obvious. I could see your concern for transmitting germs and preventing infection."

They go have sex and afterward, the woman asks the man, "Are you a doctor?"

"Yes."

"Don't tell me! An anesthesiologist! Right?"

"Yes. How did you know?"

"I didn't feel a thing."

Ophthalmology Joke: This takes place in a very exclusive private girls' school. The eighth grade science teacher, Mr. Johnson, asks, " What organ of the body, when stimulated, expands to six times its normal size? Miss Smith?"

"Mr. Johnson, I don't think that is a proper question to ask a girl of my age and social standing."

He calls on another student, "Miss Jones?"

"The pupil of the eye"

"That is correct. Miss Smith I have three things to say to you. One: you didn't do your homework. Two: you have a dirty mind. Three: someday you are going to be very disappointed."

Orthopedic Joke. A guy sees a doctor. He says, "Everywhere I touch it hurts." He touches his forehead and says, "It hurts." He touches his stomach and says the same thing. He touches his knee. Again, same thing. The doctor says, "Let me examine you." After a few minutes of poking and prodding, "Your finger is broken."

Ask any surgeon to name the three best surgeons in the world. They'll have a hard time thinking of the other two.

"Do you know the definition of "innuendo"?

"Yeah sure. That's simple"

"No. It's an Italian enema."

Plastic Surgery: During routine surgery a woman goes into cardiac arrest. After superhuman efforts and being apparently dead she miraculously recovers. During this ordeal she has an out-of-body experience in which she talks to God. God tells her she get forty more years to live and she should make the most of it be striving to be her best. From that she concludes she should improve her appearance and has liposuction, breast augmentation and a face lift. As she is leaving the hospital a bus hits her and instantly kills her. When she gets to heaven she asks God," What's this all about? You said..." God interrupts, "I didn't recognize you."

Surgery: How does a surgeon change a light bulb? They Just hold it in the socket and stand still. The earth revolves around them.

Psychiatry: How many psychiatrists does it take to change a light bulb?
Only one. But first, the light bulb has to want to change.

A man on a crowded bus a man sees a woman with grocery bags and two small children.
He gets up to give her his seat and helps her with the bags.
"Thank you. You're sweet" she says.
"I know. I'm diabetic."
Thanks to Dr. Murray Miller, an endocrinologist, for that one.

How do you tell the difference between an oral thermometer and a rectal thermometer?
The taste.

Do you have any good, clean medical jokes? If you do, please send it to me. If I include it on this list, I will give you a copy of any one of my books. Also please specify whether you want your name included as the contributor – or would like to remain anonymous. Please send jokes to Malcolm Rosenberg, P.O. Box 770793, Coral Springs FL 33077 and tell me which book you want. Simplified Arterial Blood Gases, Simplified Ventilators, Simplified Hemodynamics, Drug Calculations for Nurses Who Hate Numbers, or Making the Patients Laugh.

Q: Why are barracuda and sharks so healthy?
A: They eat fish.

Q: What is the cause of inverted P-waves?
A: Hypospadia

Q: What is the therapeutic effect of mixing Rogaine and Viagra?
A: Don King

A busy urologist's office answers the phone, "Urology Associates. Can you hold?"

Q: What did the epididymis say to the seminal vesicle?
A: "There is a vas deferens between us"

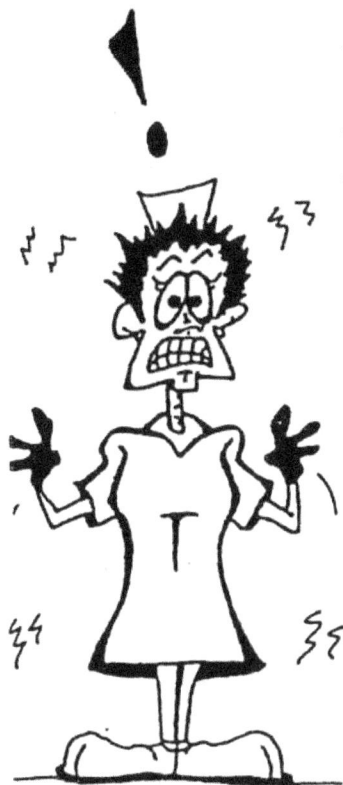
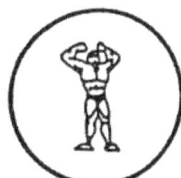 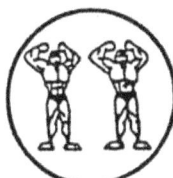 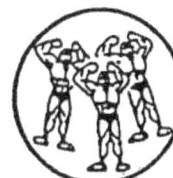
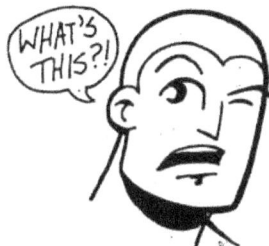
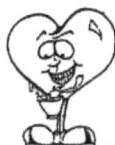 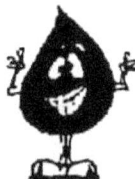 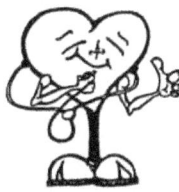 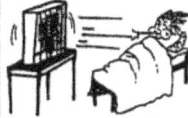 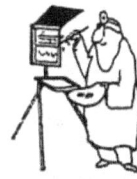 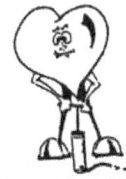

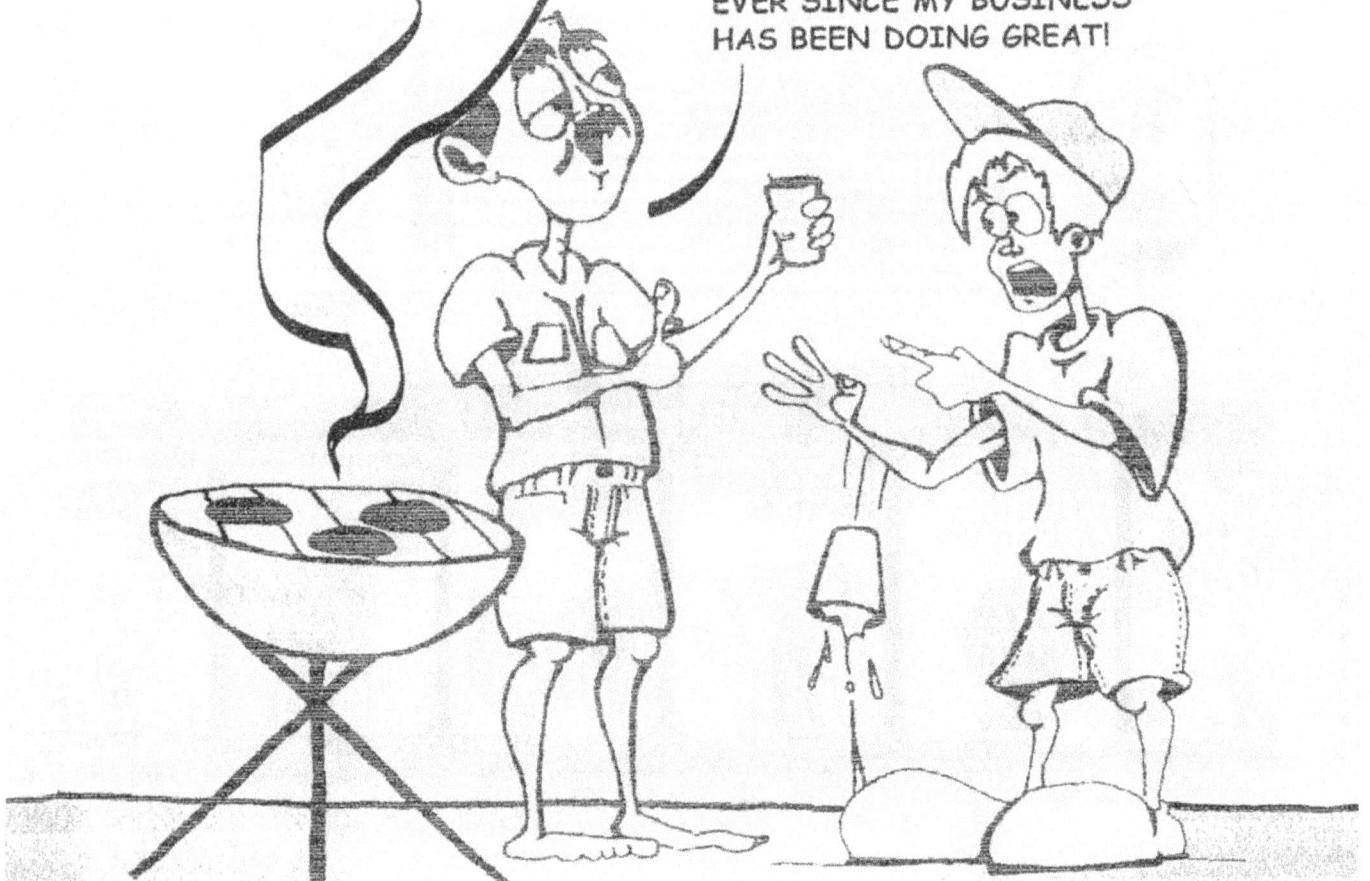

Simplified Cardiac Medications ©2001

Retail: $18.95

ISBN 0-9725483-4-3

9780972548342

0 700814 498023

7 00814 49802 3

www.ingramcontent.com/pod-product-compliance
Lightning Source LLC
Chambersburg PA
CBHW051226200326
41519CB00025B/7267